THE ANXIETY EPIDEMIC

Billie Jay Sahley, Ph.D.

Board Certified Behavior Therapist/Psychodiagnostician
Board Certified Expert in Traumatic Stress,
and Orthomolecular Therapist

Pain & Stress Publications®
San Antonio, Texas
June 2007

First Edition Printing, December 1986
First Edition Editor - Alice Evett
Second Edition Printing, January 1994
Third Edition Printing, April 1997
Fourth Edition, April 1999
Fifth Edition, October 2002
Sixth Edition, June 2007
Printed in San Antonio, TX (U.S.A.)

Published by Pain & Stress Publications®
To order additional copies, contact:
Pain & Stress Center
5282 Medical Drive, Suite 160, San Antonio, TX 78229
1-800-669-2256

Library of Congress Catalog Card Number 2007928618
ISBN: 1-889391-34-4
(13 digit) ISBN 9781889391342

Dedication

To my beloved mother, who is always with me.

*To a very special nurse
who taught me to see an eternally glowing light,
to sense hope, to find the courage to fight,
and to see the beauty of giving to mankind;
and to all RNs, members of the dedicated profession.*

*To those whose care and concern have filled my life
with the glory of love and strength.*

*To Robert Michael Benson, M.D., for his constant encouragement
to be a different kind of doctor and continue to reach out to those
who live in fear.*

*To a little boy named Scooter who is an angel in heaven now, rest
in peace.*

And to the Lord, for always lighting my path.

Acknowledgments

Not only is the sixth edition of *The Anxiety Epidemic* the story of my painful journey, but this book marks the beginning of years of research and product development in orthomolecular therapy to help those who suffer.

I have made many friends during this time, without whose help and support *The Anxiety Epidemic* might not have been written. This edition took months of extensive research, and I'd like to acknowledge the contributions of the following people.

Katherine M. Birkner, C.R.N.A., Ph.D., was there with me every step of the way with constant encouragement and help.

A special thank you to my staff at the Pain & Stress Center, for their constant support and special efforts.

My patients that teach me something new every day.

Foreword

I first met Billie Sahley some years ago when we were working at adjacent San Antonio hospitals. We soon discovered many points of mutual interest, including similar attitudes toward man's physical/mental health—or lack thereof. My reading in the field of holistic medicine was avocational; I did not realize at the time that for Billie it was a part of her professional development.

Later, our careers diverged. Billie set up her private practice as a therapist and established The Pain & Stress Clinic, and I became a book publisher. But we kept in touch, and it was natural, then, that we should collaborate when she was ready to publish her book on anxiety, its cause, and cure.

Billie's sense of mission about her work is evident in all she does. The story of her personal experience with stress, grief, and anxiety is told in Chapter I, but there is another side to this remarkable woman which is not exposed there. Deep beneath the surface, she possesses a strength of will—a determination—which has made her face every "You can't..." with an "I will!" Whether this quality was developed by her childhood trauma, or whether having such strength is what helped her survive, is moot. Her whole life is evidence of the positive result.

As something of a teenage tennis prodigy, Billie decided she would use this skill to get a college education. She was told, "You'll never make it. They don't give athletic scholarships to female tennis players." But she got the scholarship and earned her B.S. degree at the University of Texas. (She won what was then the equivalent of the collegiate national title, and later, as a pro, she was good enough to reach the semifinals at Forest Hills.)

In 1975, I saw her open an office as a Medical Marketing Consultant—the first such, I believe, in South Texas. Again she was told, "You'll never make it—and, especially, they'll never accept a woman...." But that is how she worked her way through graduate school and earned her doctorate.

This same persistence she brings to her practice today. Patients who have gone from doctor to doctor, finding no relief from their physical and mental agony, are the persons Billie reaches toward eagerly, determined that she will be able to give them the relief they have vainly sought.

There are probably other pages in her book of experiences of which I am not aware, but I know she has handled hospital public relations, prepared plans for special treatment centers, developed emergency room specifications for Class I qualification, and even been a partner in a printing company. Suffice it to say that she has continually amazed me in the years of our acquaintance—and never more than the day she remarked on the phone, "Guess who got a Ph. D. yesterday?" And I hadn't even known she was working on it.

San Antonio, Texas   Alice Evett
April 2, 1986

Contents

Charts and Illustrations

Introduction

The past twenty-one years have seen a virtual chain reaction in the public's outcry for information on the enhancement of a sound mind and body. As one result, nutrition has become a true science and is now taking its place as an integral part of health care. For years the American public lived by "you are what you eat." That has now changed to reflect the need for information about behavior, and the public is beginning to understand that "you are what you absorb."

The content of this book focuses on well-documented information and studies by leading researchers and authorities in the field of clinical nutrition, behavioral medicine, and orthomolecular psychiatry and therapy. And the understanding I offer you is the importance of nontoxic, natural substances to relieve stress, fear, anxiety, and phobias—most specifically, the proven effectiveness of gamma-aminobutyric acid, or GABA, for this purpose.

The forerunner in the use of natural substances to treat deficiency states and to produce a normal brain biochemistry is orthomolecular psychiatry. This therapy was first named and described in 1968 by Dr. Linus Pauling, a two-time Nobel Prize laureate and director of the Linus Pauling Institute. Orthomolecular psychiatry has continued to develop and provide successful models for treatment with specific nutrients in the diet and with supplements, as required. The Academy of Orthomolecular Psychiatry now includes physicians and researchers from throughout the world. The Academy has published extensive research information on amino acids, minerals, vitamins, and their effect on the chemistry of the brain.

Since orthomolecular psychiatrists rely heavily on nutrition and megavitamins, they emphasize that the human body is not naturally composed of Valium, Xanax, or any other of the tranquilizers so commonly prescribed today. The message is clear that *there is no such thing as a tranquilizer deficiency!* In contrast, amino acids, vitamins, and other nutritional factors can easily be inadequate for the body's needs, and these deficiencies can and do affect the mind and behavior.

According to the American Mental Health Association, approximately nineteen million people in the United States, alone, suffer daily from dreaded anxiety attacks, fear, panic, and phobias. They swallow annually something like 982,550 pounds of barbiturates and spend an astounding $76 billion for Valium, Xanax, Prozac, and Zoloft.

GABA (Gamma Amino Butyric Acid) is possibly the natural solution needed by these millions of sufferers! Dr. Candace B. Pert, a pharmacologist, discovered and named the GABA receptor sites in the brain and the importance of GABA in the stress-anxiety network.

Then in 2000, L-Theanine came into the picture. Theanine comes from green tea. Theanine puts your brain into an alpha state (like deep meditation). I think L-Theanine (L–T®) is equal to GABA.

I
The Story of the Wounded Healer

> You can train a cold, hostile person
> until he is 93 and he will never become a
> good "therapist." Conversely, you can
> take a genuine, empathic, warm person
> and with only a little training he may
> be a very successful "therapist."*
> —*The Natural Alternative*

Originally, my search for a nontoxic medication for anxiety was a personal one. The resolution of my own problem left me with a sense of mission to help others find drug-free relief from their own fears, phobias, stress, and anxiety.

The episode that led to my crisis and cure occurred in my twenties, when I endured circumstances of prolonged and unavoidable stress. The situation and its effects on me covered a ten-year period. The death of my mother precipitated my reaction, but the story—and the reason her prolonged illness took such drastic tolls on my mind and body—had actually begun long before.

When I was fourteen months old, a frying pan full of hot grease fell on me and I was burned over all of my face and neck. This was in the 1940s when the doctors didn't know much about burns as severe as mine. My hands and feet were tied to the crib in the hospital, and I was sprayed with tannic acid. The doctors tried to prepare my mother for what they thought was inevitable. They told

* *Psychiatry at the Crossroads,* ed. John Brady, M.D., and H. Keith Brodie, M.D.

her that since the grease was on my eyes, mouth, and all over my head, I probably wouldn't make it because of infection. If I did live, I would have brain damage.

My mother was a deeply spiritual woman, who felt that I had been sent for some special reason in her life; and she was determined that I would not die. I remember her telling me that when she came to the hospital every day, she would feed me through an eye dropper and sit with me for hours.

The healing was slow, and the disfigurement was drastic until I reached the age of twelve, when plastic surgery and skin grafting could be performed. After the operation, I lay for six weeks with my head between sandbags, unable to move. I remember vividly how helpless I felt, and how I listened for sounds to tell me what was going on around me. Then I would hear my mother's footsteps and her voice, and I would know that somehow everything would be all right. I had some fourteen or fifteen hundred stitches in my neck and it took quite a while for them to heal. The reassurance and optimism of my mother pulled me through, and made me believe that having survived this I could accomplish anything I wanted.

One of the greatest gifts given me by my mother was teaching me the power of the mind. The teaching began at a very early age, around six or seven. We would go to the church and she would always help me light a candle at the altar for my special intention. Then my mother would tell me to focus on the candle and release all my bad feelings into the flames. I remember how my eyes would become fixed on the candle flames as I sat there and listened to my mother chant the rosary. In the peaceful calm and the presence of God, we prayed together. I felt the same serenity every night after my surgery, at 6 P.M. sharp, when four nuns came into my room and chanted the rosary. My eyes would always be fixed on the candles my mother kept lit. As they chanted softly, I could hear my mother's words, "Give your pain to God, give your fear to God, His presence is here." I never asked for any pain medication the whole time I was healing; I didn't need it. My beloved mother, in her infinite wisdom, had taught me a form of self-hypnosis that I still use today! Years later, it was my turn to watch over her through her long and painful journey.

I was living in San Antonio, and my mother in Austin, when she went into the hospital for exploratory abdominal surgery. I paced the halls of the hospital for nine hours that day. I was waiting for the doctors to emerge from the operating room to tell me whether it was a minor gallbladder problem or the cancer we feared. Finally, the verdict came: pancreatic cancer. The doctors said they thought they had gotten all the cancer, but the final verdict would not be known for five years.

When I was finally allowed to go in to see her, I was warned not to show any emotion that would upset her or indicate the uncertainty of her situation. I then made the decision that she should not be told that they had found cancer. I wanted her to enjoy whatever time she had left to live in a positive way—not dreading a disease that she had always feared. I kept the candles lit for her and we prayed together.

For the next five years, I drove the eighty miles to see her three, four, and sometimes five nights a week. The stress of the situation was intensified by the recollection of the doctor's words, "You must not show any emotion; it will only make her worse." As a result, my own health began to deteriorate, and after she died, I experienced a devastating series of physical reactions to all those years of intense anxiety and depression. The stress, depression, and sadness created illness by directly affecting the functioning of my body's immune system. Compelling research data shows that the prolonged stress and grief adversely affect immune system functioning. Prior to this, I never had any problems with anxiety or accumulated stress; in fact, having been an athlete, I had always been able to let it go … through conditioned relaxation and exercise. Now I endured anxiety attacks and panic that ranged from moderate to severe, and included the entire list of physical symptoms that occur with anxiety and phobias. Many of my symptoms resembled the deterioration

I had seen in my mother's body in her last months.

Those who care for a sick loved one are hit hard and long by grief and depression. A study sponsored by the National Institute of Mental Health found 30 percent of care givers suffer from clinical depression or anxiety while their loved one is alive. Four years later 25 percent continue to suffer symptoms, while only 10 percent of non-care-giving relatives suffer depression after the death.

When I consulted numerous physicians, I was offered an assortment of tranquilizers, including Stelazine, Valium, Xanax, and Inderal (all of which I refused). Nothing more . . . no logic, no reasoning. They were never able to understand the post-trauma I was suffering, nor did they direct me to someone who could help me and explain what was happening to me and why. They could not see that I had a full-blown phobia from the *prolonged anxiety and grief.*

If I had only known then that grief felt so much like fear—the sensations were all the same. Some of the physical problems I experienced included a fluttering in the stomach, constant restlessness, tightness in the throat, fear of choking, over sensitivity to noise, weakness of muscles, lack of energy, dry mouth, a sense of depersonalization, and a tightness in my chest, so that I could not take a deep breath. I must have had five or six x-rays for this last symptom, feeling sure that something had to be wrong with my lungs. But the x-rays were always negative. Dear God, was I losing my mind? What was happening to me and why?

I had test after test, all negative. The doctors were quite willing to go on testing and offering me tranquilizers, but no one would give me any answers. I found no empathy, no sensitivity or compassion, just a constant stream of prescriptions for antidepressants and tranquilizers. The sight of hospitals brought grief, fear, and dread; and I almost became house bound. I did not want to drive, and if errands took me onto the expressway northward (the route to Austin), I would begin to shake so much I would have to pull off the road and stop. I know now that I was "playing old tapes," and that my subconscious was bombarding me for all the times I had driven to Austin under the restriction of "show no emotion."

The intense stress continued as I sat there day after day and watched them stick I.V. needles into her arms, trying to find a vein. There were no veins left. The chemotherapy that was supposed to prolong her life and stop the progression of cancer, was draining what little life she had left. All I could do was sit there and show no emotion. She would cry softly, pray for strength, and reach for my hand. As my hand touched hers, my brain and body filled with her intense pain, and I felt I could almost touch the face of death. My mind transcended to the child tied in the crib and the scorching, burning pain on my face and neck from the grease. I wanted to scream and cry, but all that I could do was pray. That was my salvation.

I took on every symptom she had—the nausea, the pain, the weakness, and especially the feeling something was in my throat. But, most of all, I became angry. The anger was not from my mother, but because I was told to show no emotion. All my depressed feelings, fears, and uncertainty began to surface in physical form. I asked questions over and over, but I was never given any answers.

Finally, the answers came, not from any of the doctors to whom I had gone, but from a wise and caring nurse. She had the experience and the compassion to know what was happening to me and to help me understand it. She, too, had walked among the flowers of fear and pain from a traumatic experience. She started me on my path to healing, and started my mind functioning. When you walk in fear, you walk alone, unless someone else who has walked the lonely path of fear reaches out and walks with you. She did, and she was always there to walk with me.

Everyday was a struggle not to allow my grief and fear to consume me. The stomach pain became so intense that I turned away from food and lived on vegetable juice and yogurt. I had already undergone one upper GI (Gastrointestinal x-ray), and nothing was found. But this time I knew that something had to be there. When it was over, the doctor who read the results was bluntly direct, "There is absolutely nothing there you have there. You do not have cancer—The only thing there is your fear!"

I was so angry I almost lost control, but I realized he had done me a big favor and made me confront the fear. Pieces began to fit into place. I remembered every time my mother would get upset her stomach would close up, and so did mine. It was our stress point, but her's developed into full-blown cancer. Here again was the mental stress, physical symptoms syndrome.

Later, further tests revealed I had a pancreatic insufficiency and I needed digestive enzymes. I had a problem digesting proteins and fats, and so did my mother. No one ever thought to check for a simple thing like digestive enzymes. One thing was very obvious; there was a genetic link to my stress points. I began taking digestive and pancreatic enzymes with every meal—dear God what a difference. There was no swelling, bloating, gas, or pain so I slowly began to eat small meals and felt better. If the fear would start, I would address it at that time. I would not allow it to take over. It was not my pain, it was pain from the past; it was not real pain. It was grief pain.

Many symptoms experienced during grief and anxiety are related. If you can find the right help (especially when experiencing for the first time the slow and tedious dying of someone close to you) . . . if things are put into perspective, then fear does not take over. Logic remains, and drugs—especially tranquilizers and antidepressants—are not needed. Drugs are not the answer.

My neurotransmitter receptors were empty because of an overload of unresolved anxiety and grief. This emptiness caused me to go through the helpless, hopeless cycle. Most significant during this period, from a nutritional standpoint I was totally depleted. No one really thinks of food during an acute grief episode. And when you also have trouble swallowing, the problem is compounded. The natural tranquilizers that the body can normally manufacture from the nutrients it absorbs were not there. My body was depleted due to the malnourished state that acute anxiety brought with it, and this condition remained as long as the anxiety did.

I never could bring myself to take any of the assortment of tranquilizers offered for anxiety, sleep, depression, stomach pains, and headaches. I felt tranquilizers would take more control away from me and cloud my thought processes. I needed a clear head to understand what I was feeling and to resolve it; let it go, and live in peace. The tranquilizers would have been the beginning of a long dependency.

Amino acids would have given me relief for each of these symptoms—but information about amino acids was not readily available. These amino acids include tryptophan, tyrosine, DL-phenylalanine (DLPA), glutamine, GABA, and glycine. Today, there are products on the market that contain a combination of amino acids that relieve the effects of acute stress. By keeping our brain receptor sites from becoming so depleted, we are no longer prone to anxiety. Even children who have attention-deficit disorder, or hyperactivity, have anxiety. Unfortunately many children and adults are allergic to milk, which is a common contributing factor to hyperactivity; yet, milk and dairy products are among the best sources of the essential amino acid tryptophan.

Knowledge is *power . . . control.* If we are to be in control of our lives, we must search for the needed information we need. My own experience—the pain, the grief, and the anxiety—presented me a challenge. Once I knew what it was I accepted the challenge and with the help of fellow professionals and friends, I did desensitize myself and finally resumed a normal life. Then I accepted a second challenge: to use my research experience to educate, inform, and help others who walk the lonely path that I walked.

Throughout my painful journey, I have seen thousands of victims of our drugged society. They never laugh, love or share; they experience only sadness. They live a very passive existence. Fear is their master, and drugs dictate what they can or will do, which is very little.

Your challenge is not to let the fear become your master. Reality is your key. You must enforce, "Nothing is going to happen." The only place it is happening is in your head. Call on your strength and follow the light to the end of your journey. At the end of your journey you will realize how much stronger you are and the ocean of fear you have crossed. *Peace be with you always and never give up hope.*

II
The Neurotransmitter Connection

Robert L. DuPont, Director of Washington's Center of Behavior Medicine, calls phobias "the malignant disorder of the *what-ifs.*"

Panic and anxiety attacks involve the brain, but are felt in every cell of the body. Certain drugs may block or relieve anxiety and panic; this strongly suggests a biochemical basis for phobia disorders. The roots of anxiety, panic attacks, and phobias lie in chemical imbalances within the brain and body. When toxic drugs block the sensations of anxiety, they disrupt or have a negative impact on important neurotransmitters, the chemical language of the brain. The brain controls every cell in the body—its commanding presence is responsible for all sensation, movement, thought, behavior, and a lifetime of traumatic memories and unresolved anxiety.

My own experience and research has demonstrated on numerous occasions, that at the time of a panic attack, some biological factors, as well as genetic vulnerability, can contribute to the physical symptoms the individual suffers. But I do not feel that biological or genetic facts are the only cause.

Many phobics can "what-if" themselves into irrational decisions and become even more helpless. Most importantly, the more control you take away from phobics, the more you feed their fear. They need control—they should make all decisions, even the smallest. The Alcoholics Anonymous theory is excellent: All you have to do is get through one day at a time. Just get through today.

Let time pass! Nothing is going to happen to you; if it were, it would have.

There is no specific single personality for an anxious person, or an alcoholic. Both perceive stress differently from the average person. Any changes in eating and sleeping habits, changes in vacations and holidays, divorce, death in the family, job loss—any of these events can cause both to perceive more stress than normal.

This perception changes the brain chemistry and depletes neurotransmitters, the chemical messengers of the brain. These chemicals send a million thought commands from one nerve cell to another. They control all feelings of fear, anxiety, anger, depression, and obsessive compulsive behavior.

In interviews with over 100 phobics whose symptoms ranged from mild, or simple anxiety, to full-blown phobias, the data given suggested the subconscious becomes saturated by past traumatic events. These unresolved events continue to draw the person back into the past—to relive the event over and over but still remain helpless to change the outcome. From this stage, the chronic anxiety often develops into multiple phobias by the time the person reaches his late twenties and thirties.

The key lies in the ability of an anxious person to realize, "It's over; let it go; let it rest in peace. I can't change it; the past is over; my control is in the present, not the past or the future!" The unresolved anxiety overloads the cerebral cortex, flooding the brain with adrenaline which starts the cycle of physical symptoms. Possibly what is now defined as faulty might, in fact, be over-saturation of the brain with adrenaline from previous years of unresolved stress and anxiety.

It stands to reason if children are subjected to a parent's constant anxiety, that they, too, will begin to feel the same anxiety. All changes in behavior alter the brain chemistry and lower the serotonin level. Take, for example, the children of alcoholics—the anxiety overwhelms them. They experience flashbacks of painful memories that seem to be imprinted into the brain through the

Nerve Cells and Neurotransmitters

A neurotransmitter is a chemical substance that transmits a message from one nerve cell (neuron) to another cell or neuron. Common neurotransmitters include serotonin, norepinephrine, dopamine, and acetylcholine.

A neuron contains a cell body, dendrites, and an axon. The dendrites carry impulses toward the cell body. The axon transmits messages away from the cell body toward the next cell. A neuron commonly includes several dendrites and one axon. Nerve cells do not link directly to the next neuron, but are separated by a synapse cleft or gap. The synaptic vesicles hold the neurotransmitters in reserve until an impulse triggers the release of these neurotransmitters so the message is transmitted to the next neuron.

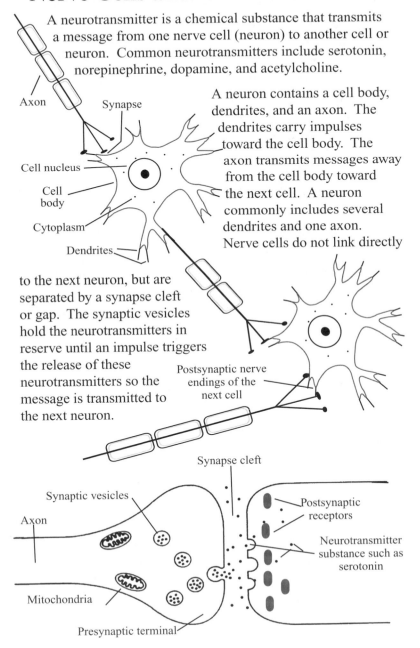

Axon

Synapse

Cell nucleus

Cell body

Cytoplasm

Dendrites

Postsynaptic nerve endings of the next cell

Synapse cleft

Synaptic vesicles

Axon

Mitochondria

Presynaptic terminal

Postsynaptic receptors

Neurotransmitter substance such as serotonin

amygdala. The amygdala is part of the limbic system, a storehouse of emotion. At any time, the amygdala can begin a bombardment of these memories—releasing fear, panic, and anxiety.

Paul's case is typical. Paul was the oldest child of an alcoholic. He cannot remember when his father did not drink. He recalls many fights that his mother and father had—mostly about the drinking. He felt a confusion of feelings, including helplessness, guilt, anxiety, fear, uncertainty, and sometimes anger. He felt trapped within the family, yet he knew he wanted help.

Paul had very few close friends because he was ashamed of his father's behavior and did not want others to know his home situation. In fact, the humiliation from his father's erratic and unpredictable behavior grew into shameful feelings about himself. He constantly tried to excel in school and in everything he did. Paul became an overachiever who was never happy or satisfied with any accomplishment. He drove himself, which produced more anxiety and kept him in a state of uncertainty. Paul was very intolerant and critical of others, often to the point of unreality.

His father's discipline varied between extremes of harsh severity or none at all, which left Paul in constant fear of what would happen or what mood his father would show next. He was never allowed to discuss the subject of drinking—this was taboo. When sober, his father was very loving, friendly, and enjoyable to be with; however, when drinking, it was as though Paul's father became a different person entirely, often becoming mean, argumentative, and abusive, mostly with words, but occasionally physically. Over the years, Paul learned to avoid him as much as possible, hoping to prevent more anxiety and conflict. He learned not to count on his father's often broken promises and lack of honesty.

Avoidance became a way of life. Paul found himself avoiding more and more activities, always anxious and fearful that something bad might happen. He withdrew and kept mostly to himself. Over the years, as this pattern grew, he developed severe anxiety and panic attacks which manifested themselves in the form of chest pains. He made frequent trips to the emergency room, but doctors never found anything wrong with his heart or chest. Finally, he sought help for the psychosomatic chest pain and learned, through therapy, how stress had conditioned his life.

The children of alcoholics constantly bring their past into the present and feel negative about the future. Letting go is not what they have seen their role models do. Parents should learn to let their children know it is OK to show fear, and it is OK to express their feelings. If children have anxiety, they should talk about it. The repressed child grows up feeling, "I can't say what I feel because it means I'm weak and not OK." Wrong! They are strong and OK!"

Norman Cousins, who wrote *The Anatomy of an Illness* and *The Healing Heart,* describes in detail how panic and fear almost caused him to accept open heart surgery that he did not need. Mr. Cousins follows the same path as my own: To educate and inform people is the greatest gift you can offer. When a person understands his body and the power of the mind, fear is no longer his master!

The greatest fear that all phobia sufferers have is that they won't be able to get help in time—before they lose control. *This control depends on the balance between the limbic system, the cortex, and the GABA receptors.* There is a great deal of evidence and research that supports the fact that GABA and other amino acids have the potential to replace many of the tranquilizers prescribed for those who suffer from anxiety, panic, and fear.

GABA is the most widely distributed inhibitory neurotransmitter in the brain. According to Michael J. Gitlin, M.D., in *The Psychotherapist's Guide to Psychopharmacology,* GABA appears to "have a very specific role to play in the regulation of anxiety." GABA, a highly concentrated neurotransmitter in the brain, primarily exerts an inhibitory effect on neurotransmission. This research was established by Doctors Tallman, Thomas, and Gallager, in 1978. There are GABA receptor sites not only in the brain, but all over the body. Forty to fifty percent of all brain synapses contain GABA. GABA plays an important role in neuronal and behavioral inhibition. The highest concentration of GABA resides in the basal ganglia, followed by the hypothalamus, hippocampus, cortex, amygdala, and thalamus. Feelings of panic, anxiety, fear, depression, anger, and grief—all dwell in the storehouse of emotion—the amygdala. Dr. Candace Pert established the importance of GABA's role in brain function.

In the last twenty-one years, I have on many occasions observed anxiety and phobia sufferers maintaining control when taking GABA and *no tranquilizers*. Many of them had, at one time, taken tranquilizers, but as time passed, they realized they had traded their anxiety for pills. Soon the anxiety crept back, and they had to take a stronger dose just to make it through the day; then a stronger pill to shut them down at night; and then wait until morning to take the next dose to stop the shakes, the fear, and waiting for the dreaded attack. Finally, someone reaches out to them and they begin to realize they want to regain control of their lives. And control does not come in a prescription bottle.

In his book, *Medical Applications of Clinical Nutrition,* Dr. Jeffrey Bland makes a very important statement regarding behavior: "Brain changes not only *can* cause changes in perception and thinking; they *do.* There are two main lines of evidence: 1) from diseases, which are known to distort the brain chemistry and cause brain symptoms, and 2) from studies of hallucinogenic drugs. A large class of psychiatric patients is characterized by changes in perception and thinking."

One of the most important aspects of Dr. Bland's book describes clinical studies brought forth by prominent researchers which establish a new era in behavior neuropharmacology. This area of medicine now presents ample evidence that nutrition can influence the production and concentration of neurotransmitters which researchers have equated with the action of drugs known to influence behavior, such as tranquilizers and antidepressants. Dr. Bland's book outlines two findings that show how vitamins and amino acids can have a direct action on the brain receptors and clinically affect changes in mood, mind, memory, and behavior.

Dr. David Bresler, author of *Free Yourself From Pain* (and my mentor in the field of pain and stress), was one of the first to publish double-blind research information on the use of amino acids such as L-tryptophan, one of the ten essential amino acids. Dr. Bresler describes the extremely important part of our brain function controlled by our serotonin level; the serotonin level is governed by our tryptophan intake. When our tryptophan intake is too low, especially during anxious or stressful periods, our serotonin supply drops, resulting in depression, anxiety, pain, hyperactivity, or agitation. Aggression is one of the most widely-recognized symptoms of low serotonin in the brain.

Dr. Bresler states that one way to cope with this serotonin deficiency is to supplement your diet with L-tryptophan. This will enhance the conversion of tryptophan to serotonin, thus resulting in a calm, relaxed, pain-free state of mind. The development of amino acid therapy promises to provide the brain and body what they need, rather than merely addressing the symptoms of the patient.

By definition, an amino acid is any large group of organic compounds which are the building blocks of proteins. There are ten which are considered essential; they are required in the diet. The body cannot create these amino acids on its own. These amino acids must be provided by the food we eat. Nonessential means the amino acids can be manufactured in sufficient quantities by the body's own tissue. Until the late 1980s, glutamine was considered a conditionally essential amino acid. This means that under normal circumstances, the body can make adequate amounts of the amino acid, but under prolonged stress, anxiety, depression or illness, the body cannot produce as much as it needs. Glutamine supplementation is necessary to prevent a deficiency. Clinical tests with glutamine demonstrated that 1,000 to 2,000 mg, per day, provide some antidepressant benefits. The essential amino acids are arginine, histidine, isoleucine, leucine, lysine, methionine, phenylalanine, threonine, tryptophan, and valine. These play a vital role in the brain's function. We have become increasing aware of the important roles of GABA, glutamine, glycine, phenylalanine, tryptophan, and tyrosine in anxiety, addiction, depression, pain, and sleep. Their roles have always been important—we just didn't know it! As information about them becomes disseminated to today's educators and throughout the media, the public is becoming aware of the dangers of dependency on tranquilizers, antidepressants, and pain pills. *Drugs do not create neurotransmitters—they only use those neurotransmitters already available in the brain.*

Stress Reaction

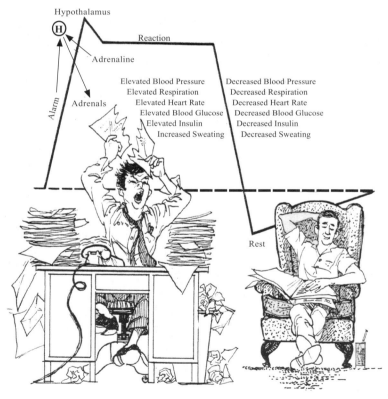

Stress in humans elicits a whole list of metabolic reactions.

III
Causes and Symptoms
Of Stress

Maria, a forty-nine-year-old housewife, felt a strange uneasiness each time she was left alone in her home. One day, as she stood at the door watching everyone leave for work and school, the uneasiness suddenly turned into uncontrollable panic. Maria began to sweat, feel dizzy and felt light-headed. She gasped for air, and her fear overwhelmed her. Her hands and feet became numb. She was sure she would die before she could get help. She managed to stagger to the phone and call her daughter to come stay with her.

That episode began a ten-year prison term for Maria. She became house bound and had to have someone with her constantly, even when she took a shower. She was seen by numerous physicians, but none were able to provide an answer for the symptoms. When I first met her and listened to her whole story, I had a feeling that whatever trauma occurred had been ongoing for a number of years.

Finally, all the pieces came together. It began when she was six years old and watched her mother leave for work every day. Maria would stand at the same window until her mother was out of sight, then wait eight long and lonely hours. She was afraid to leave the house, for she had been told that she could be hurt or killed if her mother was not there to take care of her. She never forgot that. After she got married, every time there was a crisis, her husband was away from home. Finally, it all caught up with her. She never wanted to be alone again.

After Maria and I worked through all the anger and fear, she was finally able to let go, and she began to have less fear. Self-hypnosis—especially "breathing through" attacks—and orthomolecular therapy helped strengthen her against fear. After a long year of weekly sessions, she finally enjoys having the house to herself.

Stress is a subjective and personal effect. What is stressful to one person may not be to another. People react differently to various situations. Just because something does not cause stress in others does not mean that it might not be stressful to you.

Stress attacks can come from a variety of sources, including overwork, the death of a loved one, lack of sleep, a change of residence, employment, or basic life goals—or anything which taxes you mentally and physically. Stress and anxiety use all available neurotransmitters. This usage fuels stress. Both positive and negative stresses are taxing—*even if a change is good, it can cause anxiety.*

Other sources of stress could be negative thinking habits, a high-strung or impulsive character, emotional drains, social pressures, conflicts, confusion, frustration, and boredom. Even diseases, injuries, pain, chemical or radiation exposure, and drugs can be the catalysts for stress. The warning signal for danger comes when small stresses begin to combine, multiplying their effects, leaving you overwhelmed.

The Symptoms of Stress

Much research has been done on the physical effects of stress. Stress can slowly deteriorate the health of the body.

The first level of symptoms is very slight. They can be as mild as losing interest in doing enjoyable activities, or as vague as a sagging of the corners of the eyes. Becoming short-tempered, being bored, nervous, rolling one's hands, or developing creases in the forehead can be evidence that the brain is dealing with more than it can effectively handle.

The second level of symptoms is more noticeable. Tiredness, anger, insomnia, loss of interest, fears, and sadness should be considered important warning signs that you are not managing your life well. Something needs to be done immediately to reverse the trend.

The third level of symptoms includes certain physical signs such as headache, neck ache, back ache, high blood pressure, upset stomach, strange heartbeats, tics (facial or neck contractions), and an increased tendency to become ill. These signs can be the evidence that stress is already having a serious effect on your body.

The fourth level of stress symptoms can result in actual disease. Cancer, heart disease, skin disorders, ulcers, asthma, stroke, hepatitis, kidney failure, allergies, susceptibility to infections, pain, and mental breakdown have, in some cases, been related to stress.

Many times these diseases can be reversed merely by eliminating the stress. Sometimes they can be brought on by other factors, but greatly aggravated by additional stressful conditions. Often even the condition itself creates additional stress and, therefore, aggravates the condition like the proverbial snake with his tail in his mouth.

The Physiology of Stress

The Neuroendocrine system. This system includes the pituitary and adrenal glands. Stress can affect the brain since it tells the pituitary gland to send chemicals to the adrenal glands. The adrenal gland then produces hormones which, in turn, affect the entire body. These hormones in small amounts can be tolerated well by the body and are indeed necessary, but in large amounts they can be destructive. For example, over-secretions of the *fight-or-flight* hormones (adrenaline or noradrenaline secreted during fear, rage, and excitement) can lead to a heart attack or mental breakdown. Over-secretions of the "stress" hormones (cortisone, corticosterone, cortisol), caused by long-term mental or physical effort could lead to cancer, arthritis, and susceptibility to infections.

Brain activity. If the brain cells are overworked, they can become depleted of their chemicals (neurotransmitters). Prolonged mental activity, with no chance for rest or adequate sleep, can prevent adequate time for these chemicals to be replenished and one ends up with a "dead battery." This depletion of chemicals can lead to feelings of tiredness, fatigue, "burnout," and an inability to enjoy life.

The autonomic system. This part of the brain controls the automatic functions of the body: digestion, heart rate, blood pressure, circulation, respiration, and posture. When the brain activity becomes abnormal, the electrical pathways divert into the automatic control areas of the brain. Thus, worry can cause ulcers and anxiety can increase blood pressure. (Do you have headaches, neck aches, or backaches? Your stress is going right to your back muscles. The neck and shoulders are two of the primary stress targets.)

The immune system. The immune system is depressed by high levels of the adrenal hormones. However, the immune system is affected by other factors. For example, certain "environmental stressors" such as pollens, chemicals, perfume, and even food can cause an over-stimulation of the immune system also. The chemicals contained in these factors can cause profound body reactions which we often call "allergy" or "sensitivity." This response can manifest itself with disorders such as asthma, skin rash, migraine headaches, abdominal pain and diarrhea, strange behavior, achy limbs, mouth ulcers, sinus problems, and others. Skin problems can be a direct result of emotional trauma. Eruptions often project what we cannot verbalize. Dermatologists often refer to your emotional skin; they know a sudden eruptions can result from avoiding situations that make you uncomfortable.

But, these same problems could result from "mental stress" as well. Certain thought processes and associations by some people can produce these, or similar, reactions. The challenge, then, is to discover which is actually the cause—an "environmental stressor" or a "mental" one. Often the stress is a combination of both, and each one aggravates the other:

→ Anxiety → Fear → Panic → Phobia

The key lies in control and understanding and in not allowing situations to control you. For example, if you go to a doctor, do not pre-diagnose yourself and read your own interpretation into what he or she says, for then your fear will take over. By the time you get the diagnosis, you will have already developed another set of symptoms.

At the same time, the doctor has an obligation to speak carefully when discussing your condition with you. Norman Cousins' *The Healing Heart* has the best description of the effect a doctor's words have on patients. He quotes Dr. Thomas P. Hackett, at a psychiatric convention in Montreal in 1961: "What the doctor says, how he says it, can determine [a patient's] life or death."

Fear and anxious behavior can markedly influence biochemistry. Research has shown, time and again, that the onset of illness and disease follows a cluster of traumatic events. Our behavior pattern is overtly influenced by chemical changes in the brain that include neurotransmitters that act as messengers between nerve cells. Among these messengers are serotonin, epinephrine, norepinephrine, acetylcholine, and dopamine. Because fear and anxiety alter the body's chemical balance, they directly influence the development of numerous diseases.

IV
GABA—and How It
Affects Our Behavior

Human behavior involves the function of the whole nervous system. The *limbic system,* located deep in the brain, controls behavior associated with emotions, the subconscious, and feelings of punishment and pleasure. Involved are parts of the thalamus, cortex, hypothalamus, and the amygdala.

The hypothalamus and the surrounding structures also control many internal functions of the body besides those of behavior. These "vegetative functions" include regulation of body temperature, water, hunger, eating habits, heart, and blood pressure—just to name a few.

Scientists have now established that the hypothalamus and the rest of the limbic system are especially concerned with the sensations of reward (pleasure) and punishment (pain). Electrical stimulation of certain areas satisfies or brings reward to the subject, while stimulation of certain other regions causes punishment, pain, terror, fear, a defense-escape reaction, and all the others associated with punishment. The two systems at opposite ends of the scale greatly affect the behavior of the subject. Interestingly, the combined sizes of the punishment regions in the limbic are only one-seventh as large as the reward areas.

The administration of tranquilizers, such as Xanax, to human subjects inhibits both the pleasure and pain centers, and causes a state of non-reality. Tranquilizers seem to work by suppressing many important behavioral areas, along with the hypothalamus and its associated areas in the brain.

Anger results from strong stimulation of the punishment centers in the brain. On the other hand, stimulation of the limbic and amygdala regions causes many patients to feel anxiety and fear, which is usually associated with a tendency for a person to run away. Stimulation of the pleasure or reward centers yields the exact opposite emotional behavior—the patient appears calm, relaxed, and subdued.

Probably the least understood part of the entire limbic system is the ring of cerebral cortex called the limbic cortex. This part functions as a crossover zone where signals are transmitted from the rest of the cortex into the limbic system. The function of the limbic cortex seems to be a link to the cerebral cortex for the control of behavior. The amygdala is part of the limbic system, and is involved in some of the most complex functions in the brain, including emotion and memory.

We are all aware that stress and anxiety can lead to serious malfunctions or problems in various organs in the body. For example, in experiments with animals, prolonged electrical stimulation in the punishment (pain) areas of the brain can result in severe sickness of the animal, ending in death within 24 to 48 hours. Therefore, since man is an animal, is he, too, vulnerable to this same type of stimulation of the central nervous system such as that produced by constant anxiety and stress?

Many psychosomatic disorders are transmitted from the brain to the skeletal muscle system. Anxiety, stress, depression, anger, or any other psychic state can greatly change the amount of nervous stimulation to the skeletal muscles throughout the body, and either increase or decrease the skeletal muscular tension. During periods of excitement, the general skeletal muscular tone, as well as the sympathetic tone, increases. Conversely, during sleep, muscle and sympathetic activity both generally decrease. During times of anxiety, tension, and stress, over activity of both the muscles and the sympathetic system generally results throughout the body.

The Limbic System
Medical View of Right Hemisphere

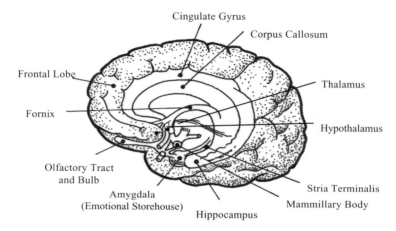

The Limbic system includes the thalamus, the hypothalamus, amygdala, parts of the reticular formation in the brain stem, and the limbic region of the cerebral cortex. Its functions deal primarily with behavior and emotions.

Some psychosomatic effects are transmitted through the body's master gland, the pituitary. Emotional turmoil can usually cause an increase in the secretion of the different glands in the body; for example, stimulation of the anterior pituitary gland increases thyroxine (a hormone produced by the thyroid), thus elevating your metabolic rate. When the metabolic rate increases, so does the adrenaline flow. This begins the anxiety cycle.

The TV series, *The Brain,* shown on PBS in 1985, gave a step-by-step description of what happens in the brain to begin the cycle of an anxiety attack. Panic or anxiety attacks occur when the amygdala, the part of the limbic system that stores and releases fear and anxiety messages, begins to release numerous signals. Concurrently, a physiological response begins to take place . . . the *fight-or-flight* syndrome as well as many others. To an anxious person, this situation of dread and fear, threatens a potential loss of control.

Stimulation of the Limbic System

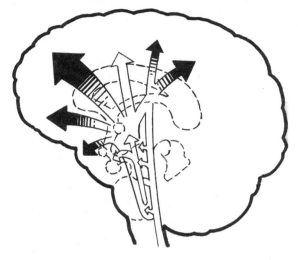

Stimulating the limbic system bombards the cortex with *anxiety* messages.

This sets up a form of the *fight-or-flight* reaction. After a period of time, the increased watchfulness and alertness that characterize these emotional states interfere with a person's sleep, making rest inadequate, eventually leading to progressive bodily fatigue and mental problems.

The autonomic nerves in the body lead directly to the internal organs. These autonomic nerves are called sympathetic or parasympathetic, depending on their function. Hyperactivity of the sympathetic system occurs in many areas of the body at the same time. The effects include increased heart rate, palpitations, and increased blood pressure, and metabolic rate. Parasympathetic stimulation generally results in more focal responses such as increased secretion of hydrochloric acid in the stomach leading to a peptic ulcer. Emotions control both the sympathetic and the parasympathetic centers in the hypothalamus, directly affecting bodily functions. High concentrations of GABA in the hypothalamus, suggests that GABA plays a significant role in hypothalamic–pituitary function.

Amino Acids' Direct Action On Brain Function

Maximum Brain Function

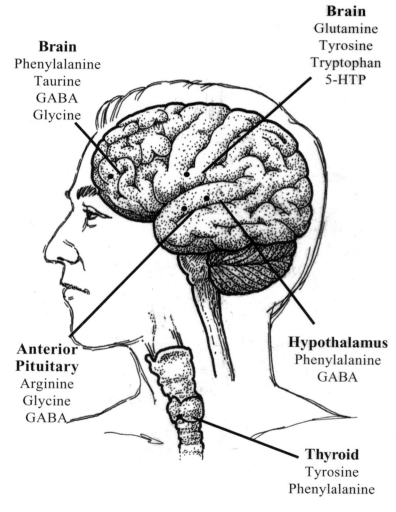

Brain
Glutamine
Tyrosine
Tryptophan
5-HTP

Brain
Phenylalanine
Taurine
GABA
Glycine

Hypothalamus
Phenylalanine
GABA

Anterior Pituitary
Arginine
Glycine
GABA

Thyroid
Tyrosine
Phenylalanine

Amino acids directly affect the brain's functions.

The unceasing alert signals from the limbic system eventually overwhelm the cortex, and the ability of the cortex and the rest of the stress network become exhausted. The balance between the limbic system and the cortex goes to pieces, often leading people into erratic or irrational behavior and fear. The ability of the cortex to communicate with the limbic system—and, in fact, the rest of the brain—in an *orderly* manner depends critically on inhibition. GABA inhibits the cells from firing, diminishing the excitatory messages reaching the frontal cortex.

GABA lowers the excitatory level of the cell that is about to receive the incoming information. If the stress, panic, fear, etc., are prolonged, GABA's ability to block the messages decreases, and finally, the process by which the signals are rated for priority breaks down and the frontal cortex is literally bombarded with anxiety messages. This breakdown is followed by a full-blown panic attack.

With the limbic system firing broadside *fight-or-flight* signals at the frontal cortex, the person's ability to reason is diminished. The effects now can include fear of dying, pounding heart, sweating, trembling, muscle tightness, weakness, loss of control, disorientation—the list is endless. Research has demonstrated that pure GABA can actually mimic the tranquilizing effects of Valium, Librium, and Xanax, but without the heavy sedated effects of these drugs. This information was first released for publication in 1982 in *Life Extension* by Sandy Shaw and Durk Pearson. Since that time, numerous studies have been published showing the successful use of GABA with anxiety-prone individuals and phobics.

Research reports demonstrate that a person who constantly experiences "what-if" type anxiety, or what is termed "anticipatory fear," has empty GABA receptors in the brain. This situation means that the brain can be bombarded with random firings of excitatory messages. It is the GABA receptor site in the brain that when adequately supplied with GABA, prevents the reception of all the random firings so that the brain does not become overwhelmed. In *Lancet,* August 14, 1982, a research report regarding tranquilizers and GABA transmission clearly stated that GABA is a major inhibitory transmitter in the mammalian central nervous system and that the agents that raise the brain's GABA concentration possess a sedative anticonvulsant property.

After the release of information on GABA in *Life Extension,* the public quickly became aware of the potentiality of GABA as an anti-anxiety formula. At the Pain & Stress Center we use a neurotransmitter formula to treat anxiety. This formula contains GABA, glycine, glutamine, B6, magnesium, passion flower, and primula officinalis. A recent survey of the medical journals reveals over 3,000 articles (case studies, clinical reports, etc.) on GABA published by researchers, scientists and therapists.

GABA and the neurons that utilize it as an inhibitory transmitter are found throughout the central nervous system. In view of our growing knowledge regarding the regulation of the physiology of the central nervous system, GABA is assuming an ever-enlarging role as a major influence over drugs, in many cases replacing them. Preliminary pharmacological and clinical data have already demonstrated the usefulness of GABA in exploring human disease.

Dr. K. J. Bergman, Mt. Sinai School of Medicine, published an extensive review in *Clinical Neuropharmacology* (1985) titled "Progabide: A New GABA Mimetric Electric Agent in Clinical Use." Dr. Bergman sums up the research and results of the clinical chemistry, the role of GABA, and the influences in the central nervous system. The most valid research published on GABA relates to anxiety.

Scott M. Fishman and David Sheehan, M.D., published a report in *Psychology Today* (April 1985) stating that as many as ten million people in the U.S. alone suffer from such anxiety or panic attacks with little or no warning and for no apparent reason. Anxiety/panic attacks can occur at any time, when a person is walking, working, resting, shopping, or driving. Sometimes, there is virtually no warning prior to the start of the symptoms.

Amino Acids for
Brain and Body Function

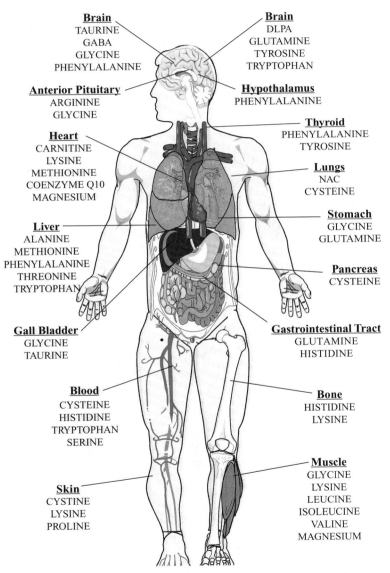

Brain
TAURINE
GABA
GLYCINE
PHENYLALANINE

Brain
DLPA
GLUTAMINE
TYROSINE
TRYPTOPHAN

Anterior Pituitary
ARGININE
GLYCINE

Hypothalamus
PHENYLALANINE

Heart
CARNITINE
LYSINE
METHIONINE
COENZYME Q10
MAGNESIUM

Thyroid
PHENYLALANINE
TYROSINE

Lungs
NAC
CYSTEINE

Liver
ALANINE
METHIONINE
PHENYLALANINE
THREONINE
TRYPTOPHAN

Stomach
GLYCINE
GLUTAMINE

Pancreas
CYSTEINE

Gall Bladder
GLYCINE
TAURINE

Gastrointestinal Tract
GLUTAMINE
HISTIDINE

Blood
CYSTEINE
HISTIDINE
TRYPTOPHAN
SERINE

Bone
HISTIDINE
LYSINE

Skin
CYSTINE
LYSINE
PROLINE

Muscle
GLYCINE
LYSINE
LEUCINE
ISOLEUCINE
VALINE
MAGNESIUM

Always add magnesium and B6 or P5'P to all amino acids.

Brain Command Center

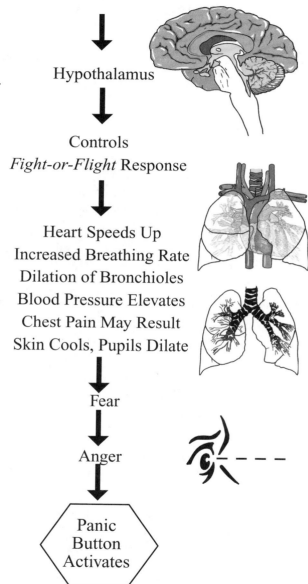

↓

Low *GABA* levels decrease serotonin levels.

Hypothalamus

↓

Low *serotonin* increases anger and feelings of loss of control.

Controls
Fight-or-Flight Response

↓

Loss of control causes anxiety and fear that triggers panic or the fight-or-flight response.

Heart Speeds Up
Increased Breathing Rate
Dilation of Bronchioles
Blood Pressure Elevates
Chest Pain May Result
Skin Cools, Pupils Dilate

Low *GABA* levels trigger increased epinephrine and norepinephrine release; that in turn, decreases logical thinking and increases heart rate.

↓

Fear

↓

Anger

↓

Panic
Button
Activates

All of this occurs in a split second.

Attacks which repeatedly occur in a particular situation begin to form a pattern. This repeated cycle causes a person to avoid that place or situation because he thinks the cause centers around that point. This is called "situational anxiety." Driving has become a major focus of situational anxiety. If you have an accident that involves injury, then fear and anxiety can be attached to driving. If you continue to withdraw, gradually the avoidance can develop into a phobia. As you begin to avoid more and more places because of the fear of anxiety attacks, you can become home bound—the only place in which you feel safe.

The variety of symptoms which characterize anxiety and panic attacks is extremely difficult for a physician to diagnose. Fear, the strongest emotion in our bodies, and anxiety and panic can all control our behavior. Some of the physical symptoms of anxiety and panic include rapid heartbeat, shortness of breath, dizziness, sweating, choking, nausea, tingling sensations, fear of dying, or chest pains. According to Michael J. Gitlin, M.D., *The Psychotherapists' Guide to Psychopharmacology*, mitral valve prolapse (M.V.P.) may be associated with panic disorder. People with M.V.P. may be at higher risk for panic disorder, while patients with panic disorder may be at higher risk for M.V.P.

NIH (National Institute of Health) reports many of the 23 million Americans who have anxiety disorders suffer in silence because they are unaware of available therapy. Information regarding the use of GABA and other amino acids is now beginning to reach those feeling trapped in a drug straight jacket, and these people are reaching out for help. GABA and other amino acids that create needed neurotransmitters hold a promising key for those who suffer from anxiety and panic attacks. GABA is responsible for keeping anxiety under control. Let me caution you; do not go buy GABA and mega dose. You can suffer side effects. Those suffering from anxiety will do anything to ease the anxiety and panic. These actions may include taking *too much* GABA. If you are uncertain about how to use GABA, consult with a therapist or nutritional consultant who understands amino acid therapy.

Published in the April, 1985 issue of *Psychology Today,* psychiatrist Ferris Pitts, at Southern California School of Medicine, found a buildup, or outpouring, of lactate in the bloodstream could cause anxiety attacks, and that an individual's behavior pattern could become disorganized. This theory was documented in Dr. Gitlin's text published in 1990.

Panic and anxiety is mediated through the limbic network. The limbic network does the integrative processing in the brain and has a direct effect on pain, fear, panic, fatigue, sleep, memory, mood, blood pressure, and the immune and endocrine functions. The limbic network is a key in selecting exactly how anxiety responses will effect the body and disrupt homeostasis.

The human body functions as an interdependent, coordinated unit—activities, actions, and reactions are directed by the brain through the vast and complex network of the nervous system. The brain, itself, is the most complex and largest mass of nervous tissue present in the body. *The brain directs all of complex activities in the body. Whatever the brain tells the body to do, it does.* Through the five senses—touch, sight, smell, taste, and hearing—the brain keeps each of us in touch with conditions and events in the world around us.

The human body performs two basic types of movement or action: voluntary and involuntary (reflex). In a voluntary action the brain calls upon the muscles or organs of the body to perform a task. In a reflex or involuntary action the senses communicate a condition or situation to the brain, and the brain responds by calling upon motor nerves to react or respond to the stimulus. In reflex actions the brain is often bypassed, and the sensory nerve may call upon the motor nerves directly, through the spinal cord, or in direct contact with the motor nerve. Reflex actions do not require thought or "brain-work" for the reaction to occur.

Researchers report that the biological roots of anxiety, panic, and nervousness lie in a tiny region of the brain near the brain stem, the locus ceruleus. Nerve fibers from this area connect parts of the brain thought to be involved in anxiety, fear, and panic attacks. The locus ceruleus comprises only a few thousand cells, but these cells produce the chemical messenger norepinephrine, which triggers the *fight-or-flight* response. GABA inhibits the activity of the locus ceruleus and slows down the firing of panic-and anxiety-related messages. Norepinephrine pathways extend from the locus ceruleus to the cerebral cortex and spinal cord, transmitting impulses that produce heightened attention.

Fear producing or traumatic situations are stored in this tiny area for playback as anxiety-or-panic-related messages. When inhibitory neurotransmitters such as GABA, glutamine, glycine, and tyrosine are depleted, the locus ceruleus, limbic, and amygdala become very active. Anxiety-related messages are constantly fired at the decision maker, the cortex, until it becomes overwhelmed.

The anatomy of memory is directed by the amygdala. Memories or uncontrollable flashbacks are imprinted into the brain through the amygdala. Flashbacks that spark the limbic system to produce fear followed by an anxiety attack come from the amygdala. *Neurotransmitters and serotonin are the keys.* When your brain is depleted, your behavior reflects it. Serotonin is the brain's master controller for all your emotional responses. When your serotonin level is low, you feel anger and aggression as well as increased pain and insomnia. Those who use prescription drugs only suppress symptoms. Their behavior is drug directed and they live in the world of prescribed addiction. Nourish the brain with what belongs there and you allow the process of healing to progress and the anxiety and fear to diminish and resolve.

The amygdala is only interested in situations that produce fear and anxiety. When the amygdala detects danger, it then changes blood pressure, heart rate, and causes a release of hormones and other responses that effect behavior. Neurotransmitters can and do effect how the amygdala behaves.

V
The Nature of Fear and Phobias

Spontaneous panic attacks—those that happen for no apparent reason—include multiple symptoms. When such an attack happens to a person, he is so overwhelmed by fear that he begins to hyperventilate and lose all reality and reason—his only thought is to get help.

John was driving on the expressway the first time he had an attack. He headed for the nearest hospital emergency room. As soon as a doctor appeared, John began to describe his feelings.

My heart is racing . . . it's banging. I can feel it in my throat . . . I know I'm missing heartbeats . . . I have a constant, sharp pain under my heart. My hands are sweaty and limp. I feel like I have pins and needles sticking in my hands (or head). I'm choking . . . I can't take a deep breath . . . my chest is so tight. I feel like I have ants crawling all over me sometimes and I want to get up and run, but I don't know where. There is a tight band, almost like steel, around my head, and there is ringing in my ears, and my vision blurs. I have diarrhea. I can't sleep . . . I wake up in the middle of the night for no reason . . . I don't know what's wrong . . . Am I going to die? I'm depressed . . . I feel dreadful. I have this terrible fear that I'm going to lose control. My mouth is dry . . . The muscles in the back of my neck are like boards. Am I having a heart attack?

Typically, the emergency room physician checked John over completely. When he was sure all was in order physically, he gave John a tranquilizer, told him he was under too much stress, and sent him home. There was no way the emergency room doctor was going to be able to convince John that his problem was emotional. This was his first encounter with the chemical straightjacket; many more would follow before he found a therapist who detoxified him (took him off tranquilizers) and began to teach him the nature of panic. He learned that spontaneous panic comes from nowhere, can last for varied periods of time, and can strike anytime. With a combination of amino acids and empathic discussions, the therapist helped John to understand and overcome his panic. John's problem was unresolved anxiety and anger.

Today, a wealth of information exists on anxiety. Both the information and the amino acids are available to physicians. They are not distributed by drug salesmen and do not require a prescription, yet amino acids are very effective. The Academy of Orthomolecular Psychiatrists has documented thousands of cases in medical journals discussing mental and physical reactions when the brain is deprived of essential nutrients. This subject is dealt with in detail in *A Physician's Handbook of Orthomolecular Medicine,* published in 1995.

Most phobics will start with a spontaneous panic attack and the severity can depend on the amount of nutrient deficiency in the brain. If alcohol has been consumed on a regular basis, the deficiencies will be more pronounced.

Agoraphobics, those with a multitude of fears, avoid public places, and focus primarily on their health. They fear a loss of control while driving, and not being able to get help in time should something happen. Agoraphobics have a lot of free-floating anxiety; while not sure exactly what they are afraid of, their behavior reflects they are afraid of everything.

Fear is the essence of anxiety! Simple or mixed phobias cause anxiety and some panic, but they focus mainly on stressful events;

e.g., traveling on expressways, driving, water, heights, flying, bridges, dentists; again, whatever they feel will take control away from them.

A fear is termed irrational when the sufferer has had ample time to learn that a situation is not as dangerous as he had initially thought, but he still persists in avoidance. The only way to conquer fear is to challenge it. Do something about it, minimize the danger, and the anxiety will go away, even though you still fear there is some danger there. That is the major reason fear persists. Anxiety is the experience of inaction in the face of dangerous situations.

Lisa was a typical phobic—firmly convinced that she had some incurable disease. But when she was examined from head to toe and told nothing was wrong, she reacted vigorously because she was sure the physician had missed something. So she went to another physician, had another test . . . still negative. Soon, she was on a steady diet of tranquilizers, dependent on them to control her fear. She was defining herself as someone too afraid to function alone. Only by not giving in to fear could she define herself as someone who was ready and able to benefit from an experience.

Tranquilizers encourage a passive approach to existence. If you are afraid of flying and take pills before or during flights, you will never learn to just relax, let time pass, and enjoy the flight. Flying represents the loss-of-control factor—that's what sets off the fear. Then why not be afraid on a bus or train?

Anticipatory fear and anxiety relate to situations of being suspended in time without knowing your future. Examples include waiting for results of a test, or traveling a plane in flight, and the middle lane of a crowded expressway. Such suspensions in time can set up a fear cycle, loss of control, and uncertainty. If worrying about the future would change it, then we should all take one hour a day to sit and worry.

There is one kind of stress which is "normal"—one caused by the result of a death in the family, divorce, job loss, etc. This kind of stress is called *exogenous* anxiety and is a reaction to unavoidable, outside situations.

Endogenous anxiety, on the other hand, comes with fear and panic—the panic attacks which can come at any time. Endogenous anxiety is thought to be biological, but there are many variables to this theory. True, the attacks are internal in origin, but if the GABA receptors are full, then the limbic system cannot bombard the cerebral cortex with anxiety. The GABA sets up a screen and slows down the excitatory messages.

Generally, a patient who is having panic attacks is likely to have underlying phobias. A person can develop a fear of a particular place or situation, and this fear is generally the circumstance that brings on the attack. Phobias can be very crippling, and the victim emphasizes the unpredictability of when the attack will occur. So he anticipates and suffers a lot of anticipatory anxiety. "What is going to happen if . . . ?" "And what-if that . . . ?" And he actually talks himself into attacks. Until I understood this in my own case, I subconsciously programmed myself daily, even to exact times of the day that the attack occurred.

These "programmed attacks" are why one might assume that panic attacks, fears, and phobias are psychosomatic in origin. Fear is the most powerful emotion of all. Fear overrides anything else within the body. What organ is stressed and is called upon when a person has fear? The adrenal glands. Putting your body under a tremendous amount of fear and stress causes the release of too much epinephrine and norepinephrine. This depletes the body of all neurotransmitters, and makes you nutritionally and emotionally a wreck.

Many patients I have treated have either been to one or two emergency rooms or have seen four or five doctors. They are usually on a whole regimen of medications which they hope will control some of their symptoms and relieve them of their anxiety. They may be taking anything from Tofranil, Prozac, Zoloft to Xanax. Some are even placed on Inderal, Ativan, Haldol, or all kinds of tranquilizers. But to date, there has been no specific drug that relieves fear as

Anatomy of A Phobia

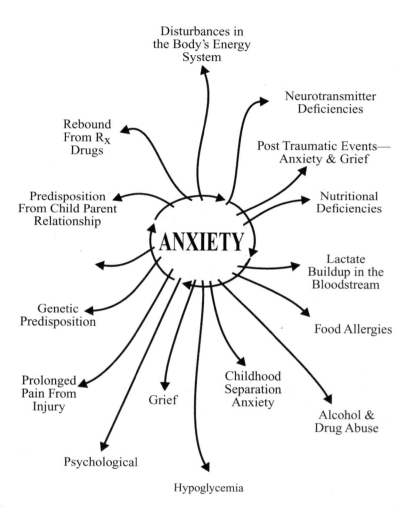

Any combination of constant emotional distress over a period
of time can cause development of acute anxiety, then a phobia.

effectively as a therapist who understands what it is you are afraid of and helps you to confront it and let it go.

Changes in behavior change the brain chemistry. Traditional medicine believes that drug therapy is far superior to talk therapy. But no study has ever shown that drugs have the same effect as an empathic therapist who understands because he or she, too, has been there and understands the face of fear and that lonely path. Research at the University of California at Los Angeles demonstrated that words can be as powerful as drugs to correct numerous errors in the brain pathways that are causing some mental disorders.

According to Peter Breggin, M.D., author of *Toxic Psychiatry*, "the modern psychiatrist may have no interest in talking therapy." This training and commitment is more likely devoted to "medical diagnosis" and "physical treatment." Dr. Breggin is an expert in psychotherapy and practices full time in Bethesda, Maryland.

One of the most unusual cases I have treated was that of a thirty-year-old male. Woody who was referred to me by his psychiatrist. His major complaint was fear of food—*any* food—unless he prepared it himself. The initial in-depth interview showed that he had multiple phobias and was agoraphobic. He was also extremely thin and suffering from malnutrition.

The food phobia started after a case of food poisoning Woody suffered from eating tainted chicken. Alone at the time, Woody had the "blind staggers" and felt as if he were dying. This precipitated an intense fear of having a recurrence.

With hypnosis, I went back with him to the age of eight years and found that his mother had been a very strong influence in his life. She constantly used negative images that projected fear. No matter what he did, her outlook was negative—emphasizing hurt, pain, and possible death. Woody's phobias stemmed from the constant bombardment of these negative images. His fixation, or phobic fear, equalled a loss of control, specifically the "helpless-hopeless" feeling. The basic focus of his fear was death.

In discussing death with me, he stated that he had experienced an intense fear of dying since early childhood. A string of accidents had reinforced the fear.

At fifteen, after a near-fatal car accident, he insisted that, despite his serious injuries, he must go home so that his mother could see him—he feared that a phone call from the emergency room would cause her to have a heart attack.

Trapped in an outside elevator, he became so panicky that he pried the doors open and jumped out. Fortunately he was only four floors up.

Another teenage trauma involved his crawling over a large area of dead bats while repairing his house. Three weeks later, he was thoroughly convinced he had rabies and was dying, despite every reassurance the doctors gave him.

Working in an oil refinery brought several major traumas; e.g., he was sprayed in the eyes with a chemical and told he would be permanently blind; he was blown off a stand by hot steam. And then came the food poisoning episode.

Woody's phobias had multiplied and diversified as he matured. He developed fear of heights, blindness, loss of control, and not getting to help in time. The episode which had indirectly brought him to me was that of waking up in the middle of the night in a state of panic—rapid heartbeat, fear of a heart attack, sweaty palms, gasping, hyperventilating, and being afraid of passing out.

Basically, Woody had been traumatized by all these events and never allowed to deal with his fears. Our process of treatment involved no tranquilizers, no drugs. Because trauma depletes neurotransmitters, Woody's brain was totally depleted and the neurotransmitters had to be restored. He was provided with a

Fear-Panic-Loss of Control Cycle

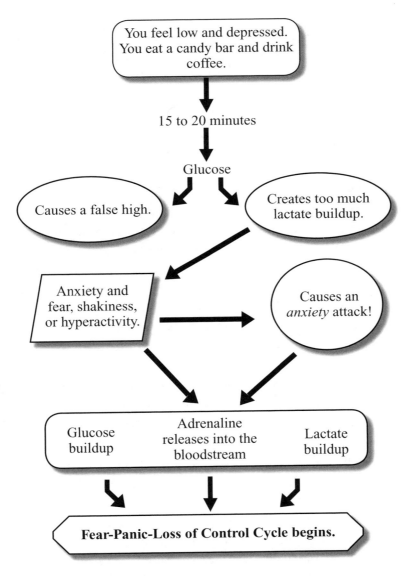

A buildup of waste products within the muscle creates lactate buildup from carbohydrate metabolism.

nutritional support program to restore his neurotransmitters and physical depletions. I taught him conditioned relaxation exercises, the "nothing is going to happen" behavior, and how to "breathe through" an anxiety attack. I told his wife the cause and character of his phobias, and she learned how to help him. In two months not only was he eating food cooked by his family, he was going to restaurants regularly with no problem. The panic attacks were gone and he was physically rejuvenated.

Many patients on their first interview come in depressed and displaying a dejected mien. Actually they have a deficiency in their serotonin level. *Serotonin plays a key role in controlling impulses.* On the other hand, a severe serotonin deficiency in children results in hyperactivity, mania, and behavior disorders; they can be irritable and overexcited—it depends on a person's individual biochemistry.

Our neurotransmitters are vitally important. If we do not get the precursors in our diet (namely, the catecholamines: tyrosine, acetylcholine, choline, serotonin, and tryptophan), the neurons cannot manufacture the neurotransmitters. They all have to be made from the precursors. The neurotransmitters control our behavior by reacting on specific receptors in the brain, such as GABA, which fills the receptor sites and keeps the limbic system from overwhelming the cortex with anxiety messages. Norepinephrine is a particular hormone needed to control problems of anxiety and depression. The presence of the amino acid tyrosine creates biological reactions which stimulate certain glands in the body to release norepinephrine and eliminate depression.

According to Dr. Alan Gelenberg of the Department of Psychiatry at Harvard Medical School, the basic cause of depression may be a deficiency of norepinephrine transmission at specific locations in the brain. A study in the effective use of tyrosine for the treatment of depression was published in the May 1980 issue, of the *American Journal of Psychiatry.*

The *Clinical Journal of Nutrition* (January 1985) states that many patients with endogenous anxiety get an infusion of sodium lactate that can precipitate panic attacks. Glucose, which increases blood lactate levels, can also induce panic attacks in people susceptible. Infusions of lactic acid sometimes can produce heart palpitations which can cause a person to fear a heart attack, and become more anxious, and set off a full-blown panic attack. Intense stress in phobics increases lactate levels, but they improve greatly after large doses of Vitamin B complex. B complex actually lowers levels of lactate. Researchers believe the improvement probably comes from niacinamide, thiamine, and pyridoxine factors in the B complex that convert lactate into pyruvic acid.

The *Clinical Journal of Nutrition* advises patients with anxiety neurosis or agoraphobia to raise their intake of magnesium and B vitamins and eliminate caffeine and alcohol. Sugar and refined carbohydrates should be greatly reduced. Fructose converts rapidly into lactate; so does sorbitol and xylitol. Reading package contents and keeping track of daily intake could save the patient a lot of anxious times. Dr. Jeffrey Bland's statement that "you are what you absorb" becomes a statement of utmost importance to anxiety and phobia sufferers.

If you would like to see the effect of diet changes on your anxiety level, eliminate caffeine, sugar, and alcohol for just one week. You will be pleased with your feeling of well being. Excessive caffeine can produce flushing of the face, palpitations, trembling, nervousness, insomnia, and addictive craving.

According to Ray Wunderlich, M.D., many hyperactive children have low serotonin, tryptophan, and B6 levels. Tryptophan apparently raises the levels of blood serotonin. Hyperactive children usually become hyperactive adults with anxiety. The deficiency from childhood carries into adult life and, more importantly, if the children are sugarholics and consume caffeine in soft drinks, they compound their own anxiety and panic just as do adults. Caffeine and sugar deplete available magnesium, which can cause an increase in the symptoms of anxiety. Magnesium is the number one stress mineral needed by the body and brain. Magnesium has a quieting effect on the central nervous system.

Prescription drugs such as Ritalin, Prozac, and Xanax do not create neurotransmitters. They only use those available. For information on the ineffective, but addictive, properties of Xanax, Prozac, and Halcion, see *Consumer Reports*, January 1993. Joe and Teresa Graedon reported in their column *in The Peoples' Pharmacy*, October 1989, "Xanax is one of the most dangerous and commonly prescribed minor tranquilizers in the U.S." Reports show it has been associated with confusion, paranoia, depression, and hostility.

Panic Attack or Allergic Reaction?

Allergies do not just cause the sniffles and itchy, watery eyes. Few physicians and even fewer patients know that ordinary allergies—food, airborne, or chemical sensitivities, can cause psychological reactions. Symptoms range from mood swings and depression to full-blown panic attacks.

Since panic attacks are no longer uncommon, most physicians suspect a psychological problem, when the culprit could be a food allergy or other sensitivity that won't show up in standard allergy tests. Many times during my personal episode I experienced what I thought was a panic attack . . . rapid heart beat, shortness of breath, irritability, and tension. These sensations continued even after I was on a good orthomolecular program, and my grief and depression resolved for the most part. Determined to stop any of the old feelings, I began to research what could possibly be the cause of physical symptoms I was experiencing. I focused on the accelerated heartbeat in relation to allergic reactions because I knew I developed a sick headache and rapid heartbeat from certain odors. The formaldehyde fumes from a new carpet in my home were literally driving me crazy every night. I was experiencing a chemical reaction that produced the physical symptoms.

Then, as I went through the symptoms of food allergy, I realized what I thought to be a panic attack was, in fact, an allergic reaction to milk. I always had digestive problems with milk, and so did my mother. At that time I thought the best thing I could eat was yogurt, and did so regularly. Because of my reactions I knew it had to be a severe allergy, so I stopped consuming all dairy products. Forty-eight hours later the symptoms stopped.

The tendency to develop food allergies is increased if the intestinal lining has been damaged for any reason. One example of this is a person who has regular diarrhea, or irritable bowel syndrome. The intestinal wall becomes porous, then loses some of its normal protective lining or immune barriers.

Oddly enough, the foods you crave the most are the ones to which you could have a food allergy. If you think you could be allergic to one or more foods, there are available tests that only require one blood draw for accurate results. A quick way to check, when you are having the symptoms, is to take an *Alka Seltzer Gold*. Alka-Gold neutralizes food reactions and the symptoms stop in minutes. Make sure you use only the *Alka Seltzer Gold* because of its special formula.

The following lists some of the mental symptoms that can be related to food allergy: aggression, agitation, anxiety, compulsions, confusion, crying easily, depression, distraction, excitability, fear, feelings of unreality, impatience, insomnia, irritability, jumpiness, lack of concentration, mental confusion, nervousness, panic, rage, restlessness, sensitiveness, slow thought processes, talkativeness, temper, and tenseness. The following lists of symptoms can be related to an allergic reaction to cow's milk: dark circles around the eyes, abdominal distention, abdominal pain or stomachache, constipation, diarrhea, gas, indigestion, asthma, nasal congestion, sinusitis, sore throat, stuffy nose, wheezing, behavioral disorders, cardiac irregularities, headache, hyperactivity, irritability, musculoskeletal discomfort, excessive sweating, and tension.

I've had several hundred patients come to the Pain & Stress Center who described these symptoms in detail. Over half of them had seen a physician and, you guessed it, they were given Xanax or Ritalin instead of treatments for food and airborne allergies. We tested them and withdrew the offending foods from their diets for at least 30 days. The next step was a food-rotation diet.

Allergy sufferers respond to a balanced hypo-allergenic supplement program. The amino acid, tyrosine, is very beneficial. Tyrosine helps fortify the immune system because one breakdown product of tyrosine is epinephrine. Environmental medicine doctors use tyrosine to treat acute episodes of allergic reactions. If you suspect this could be one of your problems, keep a food diary and note how you feel after you eat certain foods. If your anxiety is food-allergy related, your pulse rate often increases, causing you to become very aware of your heartbeats and even experience shortness of breath. Keep a diary of the foods you eat. The diary can help you establish a pattern of possible offending foods. Two excellent resource books are *Tired or Toxic* and *Wellness Against All Odds* by Dr. Sherry Rogers. These books will help you greatly.

For those of you who have airborne allergies, you need at least 5,000 mg of Ester C daily in divided doses. Ester C has a pH of 7.0, which means it is as neutral as distilled water, and you will not experience any adverse side effects from Ester C that you might have with regular Vitamin C. Ester C is safe for children and infants.

VI
The Orthomolecular Approach to Treatment of Anxiety

In my work and research with people who suffer from anxiety, fear, panic, and phobias, one factor has surfaced continually: *anxiety has a direct effect on the body's physical/physiological symptoms.*

In Dr. Harold Gelb's book, *Killing Pain Without a Prescription,* he stated that muscle tension causes most of the pain suffered in this country. Dr. Gelb showed that an astounding seventy to eighty million individuals suffer some type of muscular pain. Why? The precipitating factor in most cases is stress and their inability to cope with it.

Each of us begins to practice our coping skills as early as age four or five; the ways in which we do or do not handle stress will carry into our adult lives. Each person's ability to handle anxious/stressful situations depends on an extensive list of factors, including family environment, predispositions, child-parent relationships, a lifelong challenge of stress conditioning, as well as our ability to be influenced by chronically ill or negative individuals around us. Factors that cause the damage are multiple, complex, and chronic.

An example of the situational anxiety that may develop from childhood through adulthood is the case of the offspring of an alcoholic, such as Paul in Chapter II. Exposed day in and day out to his father's illness, Paul experienced loss of control, anxiety, fear, and a constant feeling of uncertainty. As a child and then as an adult, he suffered from a continuous anxious state. Imagine the condition of the chemoreceptors in his brain; is it not possible that the day-in, day-out fearful state damaged or made the chemoreceptors oversensitive and misfire? This misfiring or traumatic occurrences of various kinds, would create panic from fear whenever flashbacks of his childhood occurred, especially if one or both parents were physically abusive.

Considering that alcoholics are malnourished, the condition of their children would probably not be average. Since every cell in our body changes completely every six months, what we absorb determines our state of health. If alcoholics do not receive, or are unable to absorb, the necessary nutrients, essential amino acids, and minerals, they—and their children—will stay in a minus state of nutrition, predisposing them to both physical and emotional illnesses. According to Roger J. Williams, in *Nutrition Against Disease,* "An alcoholic should supplement his diet with a good assortment of minerals and vitamins—even amino acids," since his years of drinking have typically caused malnourishment.

The tranquilizers so often given to alcoholics' children, to help them cope and sleep, are nothing more than a sugar coating of the problem or possibly the beginning of their own addiction. The tranquilizers simply cover up the symptoms, but do not remove the cause.

In *Brain Allergies—The Psychonutrient Connection,* by William H. Philpott, M.D., and Dwight Kalita, Ph.D., the authors state that toximolecular psychiatrists (those who use drugs or synthetic substances not normally found in the human body) may think they are practicing scientific medicine, but they are not. Even though tranquilizers manage to control psychiatric symptoms, the underlying disease process initially responsible for the symptoms usually remains unchecked. Drugs only treat symptoms.

Linus Pauling, when defining "orthomolecular medicine," said that the treatment of disease is a matter of varying the concentration of substances (i.e., the right molecules: vitamins, minerals, trace elements, hormones, amino acids, enzymes) normally present in the human body. Through regulation of the concentration of chemical molecules, orthomolecular medicine aims to achieve and preserve

Mechanized, Urbanized, Unbalanced Individual

- Over-Rested
- Over-Protected
- Over-Fed
- Under-Exercised
- Under-Disciplined
- Over-Stimulated
- Under-Released

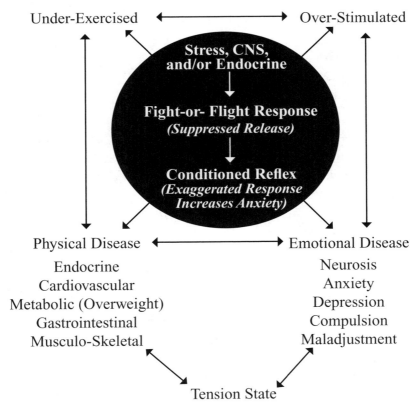

Under-Exercised ⟷ Over-Stimulated

Stress, CNS, and/or Endocrine

↓

Fight-or- Flight Response
(Suppressed Release)

↓

Conditioned Reflex
(Exaggerated Response Increases Anxiety)

Physical Disease ⟷ Emotional Disease

Physical Disease	Emotional Disease
Endocrine	Neurosis
Cardiovascular	Anxiety
Metabolic (Overweight)	Depression
Gastrointestinal	Compulsion
Musculo-Skeletal	Maladjustment

Tension State

Hypokinetic Disease by H. Kraus and W. Raub, Charles C. Thomas, Publisher, documents the above illustration.

optimum health and the prevention and treatment of disease.

Many physicians are unfamiliar with the orthomolecular approach and know only the drug or toximolecular approach. Dr. Philpott states that "drugs are chemical substances which, even if given singly, radically alter man's metabolic machinery and many times interfere with normal vitamin, mineral, amino acid, and enzyme activities in the body. Nutrients, on the other hand, working as a team, act constructively as building blocks for life in general; without them, human life could not exist. Life can exist without drugs!" A much better quality of life exists without drugs.

Abram Hoffer, M.D., Ph.D., an orthomolecular psychiatrist, warns that he has seen many hyperactive young children placed on symptomatic drug therapy such as Ritalin. This type of therapy brings hyperactive symptoms emotionally under control, but later the patient degenerates further into adult schizophrenia. The adult schizophrenia results because the underlying metabolic cause remains untreated.

Toximolecular medicine requires only one thing from its patients—that they continue to take their drugs or tranquilizers. To think that these patients on drugs often have to pay an extremely high price for their symptomatic relief is disturbing; they run the statistically high risk of becoming permanently incarcerated and/or controlled by their chemical straightjackets.

Hoffer and Walker in *Orthomolecular Nutrition* offer the following summary.

> "Every tissue of the body is affected by nutrition. Under conditions of poor nutrition the kidney stops filtering, the stomach stops digesting, the adrenals stop secreting, and other organs follow suit. Unfortunately, some psychiatrists labor under the false belief that somehow brain function is completely unaffected by nutrition. It seems that many psychiatrists and their parapsychiatric colleagues such as psychologists and social workers consider the brain is not an organ of the body that needs nourishment."

There is no such thing as a tranquilizer, antidepressant, or stimulant deficiency. Drugs cannot cure pain, stress, anxiety, depression, or grief—they can only block these symptoms.

Biochemical Imbalances

"At present there are no known biochemical imbalances in the brain of typical psychiatric patients—until they are given psychiatric drugs. It is speculative and even naïve to assert that antidepressants such as Prozac correct underactive serotonergic neurotransmission (as serotonin biochemical imbalance). Since these imbalances have not yet been identified, it makes no sense to give toxic drugs, including the currently available antidepressants and neuroleptics, all of which grossly impair brain function."*

*Excerpt from *Brain Disabling Treatments in Psychiatry* by Peter Breggin, M.D.

Symptoms of Anxiety

The following lists some of the anxiety-fear-panic-phobia symptoms that have shown improvement with orthomolecular therapy.

1. Feeling a loss of control
2. Think you're going insane
3. Feeling light-headed, faint
4. Unsteady legs
5. Having difficulty breathing—unable to take a deep breath
6. Fearing a heart attack
7. Pounding, skipping, racing heart
8. Experiencing a constant fear of dying
9. Feeling tingling in lips and fingers
10. Experiencing stomach pain, diarrhea, constipation, nausea
11. Sweating, excessively even when cold
12. Experiencing headaches, neck and shoulder pain
13. Experiencing low-back pain
14. Feeling tender headed
15. Feeling tired, weak, no energy
16. Feeling as though you are outside your body
17. Experiencing mood and emotional swings
18. Experiencing insomnia
19. Sleeping restlessly with or without nightmares
20. Experiencing an inability to relax
21. Feeling anxious, tense, and/or restlessness
22. Having depressing or negative thought patterns
23. Needing to have someone near you constantly

24. Having a rush of panic or fear, for no reason
25. Fearing crowds, breathing with difficulty
26. Eating emotionally, food won't go down
27. Muscle twitching, muscle spasms
28. Experiencing an inability to remember
29. Staying home
30. Having dry cotton mouth
31. Experiencing blurred vision
32. Feeling mental confusion
33. Experiencing flushes (hot flashes) or chills
34. Having choking sensations
35. Experiencing chest pain
36. Having numbness and tingling of fingers and lips
37. Fearing the dark
38. Perspiring more than normal
39. Flushing of the face
40. Constantly passing gas (indigestion)
41. A feeling food won't go down
42. Experiencing muscle spasms
43. Never feeling full (bottomless stomach)
44. Experiencing muscle stiffness
45. Experiencing tension headaches

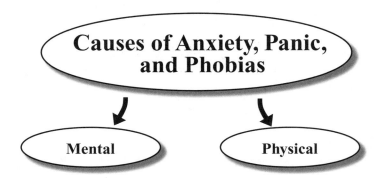

Causes of Anxiety, Panic, and Phobias

Mental   **Physical**

Nutritional Deficiencies
↓
Neurotransmitter Deficiencies
↓
Post Trauma
↓
Unresolved Anxiety
↓
Psychological Conflicts
↓
Grief
↓
Food Allergies
↓
Prolonged Pain From Injury
↓
Biological Factors
↓
Childhood Separation Anxiety
↓
Rebound Drugs
↓
Hypoglycemia
↓
Lactate Buildup in the Bloodstream
↓
Alcohol & Drugs
↓
Disturbances in the Body Energy System
↓
Genetic Predisposition

Brain Pathways of Mental Distress

The neurotransmitter GABA modulates anxiety in the brain. High concentrations of GABA receptors are found in every cell of the brain and body. GABA affects processes involving motor coordination (cerebellum), information retrieval (hippocampus) and cognitive processes (cerebral cortex).

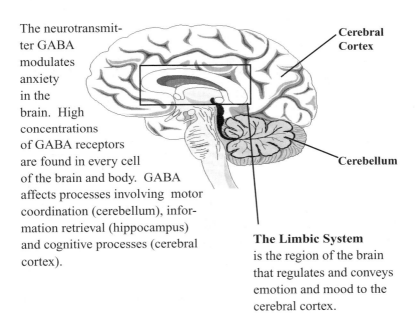

Cerebral Cortex

Cerebellum

The Limbic System is the region of the brain that regulates and conveys emotion and mood to the cerebral cortex.

Anxiety, panic, and grief deplete the brain of amino acids which are the precursors to inhibitory neurotransmitters in the brain. The neurotransmitters are the chemical language of the brain. The amino acids GABA, glutamine, glycine, tyrosine, taurine, and tryptophan are very important to those who suffer anxiety and fear, and should be taken on a daily basis. GABA, glutamine, and glycine are for relieving anxiety. Tyrosine relieves depression. Taurine assists the skeletal muscle and central nervous system. 5-HTP improves sleep. Melatonin also can be helpful for restful sleep. Mag Link (magnesium chloride) is essential to alleviate insomnia and promote restful sleep. Amino acids are an extremely important part of the healing process.

VII
Solving the Puzzle—
The Healing Begins

Empathic Understanding—This kind
of understanding is sharply different from
the usual evaluative understanding,
which follows the pattern of, "I understand
what is wrong with you." When there
is a sensitive empathy, however, the reaction
in the learner follows something of this
pattern: "At last someone understands how
it feels and seems to be me, without
wanting to analyze or judge me. Now I can
blossom and grow and learn." This is
the very special way of being with another
person which is called "empathic."

Carl Rogers
A Way of Being

Dr. Rogers sums up what I consider the most important factor
in reaching and helping a person who has suffered for many
years. A therapist's own empathy is the best qualification. Through
this process he or she is able to put a face on the patient's fear for
the first time and light up a part of the sufferer's life that has been
shrouded in dread and darkness. Empathy creates a bond between
the therapist and the patient, especially when the therapist does not
identify him or herself as an authority figure or become judgmental.
That special empathy is part of a *wounded healer*—one who has
suffered and walked from the face of fear and darkness into light

and understanding. Choose one who walks *with you,* not in front of you.

Dr. Rogers demonstrates the potential for success in reaching out. "When the other person is hurting, confused, troubled, anxious, alienated, terrified, or when he or she is doubtful of self worth, uncertain as to identity . . . then understanding is called for. The gentle and sensitive compassion offered by an empathic person provides illumination and healing. In such situations deep understanding and sharing is, I believe, the most precious gift one can give another."

Implement a Multi-Dimensional Approach to Desensitization and Healing

A large part of moving through your anxiety, fear, and phobias means accepting responsibility for *yourself and only yourself.* You must choose, make hard decisions, accept consequences, get rid of excuses, and blame no one; and, too, explore all natural resources for mind and body—listening to and becoming aware of your body's needs, as well as its rejections.

The subconscious can handle only so much storing of the negative, only so many times that you say, "I can't handle that . . . I can't deal with that." There comes a time for dealing, and if you don't stop and deal with it now, when will you deal with it? When a person lacks the capacity to act on the basis of his own power, he sets himself up to be threatened by every new situation which requires autonomous action.

Another strong factor enters the picture . . . *repression.* Repression of needs, true feelings, anger, and self-esteem. Repression decreases autonomy and increases helplessness and inner conflict.

Anxiety and hostility are interrelated—one generates the other. First, anxiety gives rise to hostility. This relation can be understood in its simplest form; anxiety, mixed with hostility, creates helpless isolation and conflict—all exceedingly powerful experiences.

Other powerful and painful emotions relate to the loss of self-esteem, loss of confidence, and the feeling that you can't do anything right. All those things depend on you, *your* judgment. Whatever your own concept of anxiety is, it is just that—your own concept. Anxiety, fear, and phobias are all your own. Unique to you, they all have your own personal characteristics. Anxiety reflects the kind of personality you have developed from infancy and childhood, through your adult life, right up to today.

At times, in childhood as well as maturity, when anxiety cannot find a release, it surfaces in physical form. The result may be an outbreak of hives, a migraine headache, neck pain, or even sudden weight gain or loss. Arthur came to me twenty-four hours after an outbreak of hives caused by an anxiety attack. He felt helpless, but he was repressing this emotion. He did not see the relationship between the anxiety and the hives.

Anxiety, stress, fear, and pain will always attack your weak spots, and they know where they are—migraines, backaches, headaches, sweating, nightmares. Don't fight it. Understand it. Deal with it for what it is . . . an emotional outpouring. To give in to it or to refuse to see what it is trying to point out is to let it become much stronger and gain that much more control.

Acknowledge the panic, the anxiety; then sort it out and look at it. Take the positive, take the negative, and examine them from both sides. It can't grow if you sort it out . . . if you deal with it, if you are in touch with it. "I know what's happening," you tell yourself, "I know what's going on."

Confront fear, confront anxiety. "Why am I afraid of the situation? What do I think is going to happen? What am I anticipating? What has happened in the past that I think might happen now? Are you in the past? If you are, that is why you feel anxiety; you don't belong there. Why do I feel I have no control?" If you stay in the present, you will have control.

Relax, let time pass; don't hyperventilate. Understand what is going on inside of you. Remember, *a relaxed muscle cannot have an anxiety attack.*

Don't run, let your feelings come. Don't fight the feelings of panic. When you feel the panic mount, relax, take a deep breath, always inhaling through your nose and exhaling slowly through your mouth. Reinforce: "Nothing is going to happen! I'm okay!"

The reality within you is a great asset and your conscious mind waits for you to say, "Wait a minute; I'm going to bring this thing into perspective." Maybe you can't drive on the expressway right now, but the longer you sit there and think about it, the more fearful you become. Negative thinking produces negative action. Fear thrives on negative feelings.

In helping phobics work through panic and anxiety, I have found that teaching them self-hypnosis is very effective. Since all hypnosis is self-hypnosis, or an altered state of consciousness, you can use it to project yourself through fearful situations and remain relaxed.

The easiest way to get into an altered state is to take a few slow, deep breaths, let your eyes close, and count slowly from ten to one. When you open your eyes you should be completely relaxed. (See Self-Help chapter for procedure.) With practice you can use the self-hypnosis to work through many difficult situations. When I learned this procedure, it became one of my main keys to conquer fear. The more I went through it in my mind, the less anxious I became.

As a practical example—I use it today when I go to the dentist. In the past, I had an unpleasant experience when a dentist almost let me gag on cotton, and the memory left me with a fear of choking. I told my current dentist of the episode, and he helped me overcome this irrational fear. When I learned the technique of self-hypnosis, I decided to avoid the hanging lower lip which results from a shot of Novocaine, and learned to put myself into a deep state and feel no pain. The system is easier on me and on the dentist. Now I send him many anxious and fearful patients, and he is wonderfully successful with them. If you have a problem having dental work done, take the time to explore your problems and your dentist. Dental phobias come from a fear of loss of control, but an understanding dentist, staying relaxed, and the Anxiety Control 24® formula can make a big difference. John Moore, D.D.S., has certainly made a major difference in my life.

Projecting yourself successfully through a situation reinforces the assurance that nothing will happen. The anxiety lasts only for minutes; control comes with your ability to relax and remain relaxed. Fear and relaxation don't mix. And each successful experience makes the next easier to achieve.

Let me go over again a few constructive ways in which you can handle anxiety, instead of letting it handle you. The key is an expansion of awareness. Don't let the conflict get started. Restructure your goals if you have to, make allowances if needed, but don't give in and be unrealistic and say "I can't do it." You are the one in control. You achieve what you believe you can achieve. You achieve what you want to achieve. And when you have achieved something, the feeling within you is projected, and what is projected becomes the confidence and the self esteem that you need to overcome the anxious feelings.

These are all therapeutic ways of dealing with yourself, a self you can continue to improve, or a self that you can allow to become stagnant. Your life is yours. You need not be controlled by fear. People talk about someone hearing a different drummer . . . you may not feel the same way somebody else does about a situation. That's OK. You have a right to feel differently.

Create your own mountain, and when you get to the top of that mountain, you will not find any anxiety or fear. Leave the chronic apprehensiveness at the bottom as you climb. It doesn't matter if the mountain is very small in the beginning . . . each time you climb it, it will become bigger and you will become stronger. As your growth continues, so will your happiness. Growth and happiness increase one's awareness; use it to reduce anxiety and fear to normal levels, and then use the normal anxiety to stimulate your own awareness.

Another way of saying it is that anxiety is a signal that something is wrong in one's personality or relationships. You may view anxiety as an inward cry for resolution—resolution of a problem that you've been carrying—of unresolved anxiety. The cause, of course, can have an infinite number of sources.

The anxiety may be the result of some misunderstanding between you and your mother or father, or with a friend, lover, or spouse, which can be resolved with authentic *communication* with the other person. Open communication can resolve a surprising number of problematic or frightening situations. Our refusal to communicate . . . our fear to communicate . . . our lack of knowledge of how to communicate . . . our fear of telling someone how we feel so that they can better deal with us and we can deal with ourselves and others—*these form* the basis of our relationship problems.

Or, perhaps, an expectation of one's self at a stage of development when the expectation cannot be realistically achieved, creates anxiety. If you feel that you are not able to accomplish what you should, then you become anxious and can go into avoidance. Anxiety can be triggered by an awareness of the limitations of your life—limitations of one's intelligence, relationships, unavoidable loneliness, or some other aspect of your life. In these cases, anxiety can take the form of mild or intense dread.

The intensity of these situations can, of course, vary. Dread may be simple undercurrents of apprehension, or graphic imagining of something about to happen to us. In these cases, we tend to use a tremendous amount of negative thinking to deal with the fear, or we go into complete avoidance and perhaps even become house bound. This is our way of not confronting—of refusing to face the problem. Rejection and fear of rejection can and do cause us to avoid dealing with a problem, especially if it involves our family.

One of the most thoroughly phobic patients I have ever worked with was Sister Karen, a fifty-one-year-old nun, high school teacher, and counselor. She was an introvert, a workaholic, and an agoraphobic. She began to develop phobias as she continued to internalize her anger, fear, and depression. There were several bouts of physical illness due to extreme fatigue—both physical and mental. She had been hurt emotionally numerous times and was never able to deal with it. Her anxiety began to deepen and the phobic physical symptoms continued to take control.

Here is the incredible list of fears she presented at a session.

1. Fear of death
2. Fear to let others know what's happening inside of me
3. Fear of not being accepted
4. Fear of being useless
5. Fear of being dependent
6. Fear of being incapacitated
7. Fear of going blind
8. Fear of what others think about me
9. Fear of being in an accident
10. Fear of being late
11. Fear of knowing who I really am
12. Fear of not being strong enough
13. Fear of not being able to handle family death
14. Fear of what may happen to my brother in his marriage
15. Fear of my oldest sister
16. Fear of authority
17. Fear of hurting others
18. Fear of appearing before a large group
19. Fear of giving my opinion
20. Fear that my way of sharing may be all off target, or that I do not explain myself intelligently
21. Fear when someone calls me aside to say something
22. Fear at times when called to the phone
23. Fear of becoming very weak and collapsing somewhere
24. Fear of going out of my mind
25. Fear of being in a psycho ward
26. Fear of not leaving others free—of getting in their way
27. Fear lest people will not be/are not open and honest with me

28. Fear of not doing a good job
29. Fear of being in church (in a large crowd) for a long service; needing to sit on the end of the bench
30. Fear of the future
31. Fear of losing my vocation
32. Fear of people not keeping my confidences

The first step in helping this woman was reality therapy—and getting her to relax and let her feelings out. She needed reassurance that it was OK to say, do, or be whatever she felt. She had a tremendous fear of drugs or any loss of control.

A nutritional evaluation established she was physically depleted to a dangerous degree. Nutritional supplements were suggested and they proved very beneficial.

After six months of therapy, Sister Karen began to recover and her personality strengths came to the surface. Now she knows who, what, or how—it's OK to be who you are. I cannot help feeling that a major influence in this case was the fact that I could understand the depth of her pain because I had once walked the same paths, felt the deep hurt, and wondered what the Lord had in store for me. It had come to me, finally, that my purpose was to give of myself, to help others, but not to lose my identity.

Sister Karen had been sent down the same path. Watching her become enriched by life has reinforced my convictions of why I am on this earth. Today, Sister Karen is like no other, and her presence is known and felt by all others in a positive beauty that radiates when she enters a room.

Understand Your Body Biochemistry

An ordinary day of physical exercise is a pleasant experience which puts you in a happy mood. The epinephrine (adrenaline) that goes to your heart is normal. But when you are in a situation of extreme anxiety or panic, the increase in the amount of adrenaline, plus sudden infusion of more hormones known as catecholamines (adrenaline), can disrupt the rhythm of the heart. If the constant stress on the heart continues, it could rupture the heart muscle fibers. If you have a magnesium deficiency, then your problem will get worse. The heart needs magnesium to nourish it (see Nutritional Medicine chapter for information on magnesium).

If you are relaxed and without anxiety and fear, you will be able to do whatever you enjoy. The power of the mind (projecting calm, relaxation, and peace, such as in self-hypnosis), programs the brain and hormones and endocrine system. You are your own protector. *Uncertainty is the number one feeling which causes anxiety to become a panic state.*

Uncertainty → Anxiety → Panic → Fear → Phobia

Biofeedback Therapy

Biofeedback training excellently mirrors the changes in your body. This information tells you what physical changes are happening to you under stress. With biofeedback training you can learn how to slow down your heart and realize what a state of total relaxation is—in contrast to an anxiety attack.

Biofeedback uses instrumentation to mirror psychophysiological processes of which the individual is not normally aware and which may be brought under voluntary control. Biofeedback provides the person immediate information about his own biological conditions, such as muscle tension, skin surface temperature, brain wave activity, galvanic skin response, blood rate, and heart rate. This feedback enables the individual to become an active participant in the process of phobic desensitization.

Biofeedback involves the use of specialized instrumentation. The equipment may be as simple as a thermometer or as sophisticated as an electroencephalograph—an electronic device which measures brain wave patterns. The most important feature about the instrumentation, no matter how simple or complex, is that it tells the individual about the measurement which it just made. This important, immediate feature distinguishes biofeedback from other techniques that teach "relaxation" or "alpha control," but which do not involve feedback of actual physiological changes.

Hold a small thermometer between your finger and thumb, and think about your fear. Your temperature will drop and your hands will become cold. Now begin to breathe deeply and slowly and let go of the fear, and watch your temperature rise. That is how fast your body records changes of fear and anxiety. Self-hypnosis with biofeedback is one of the best ways to train yourself to control stress and anxiety.

The use of biofeedback instrumentation provides a means to an end. As a very useful learning technique, the individual can learn better control over certain psychophysiological processes. The end result is that you can exercise this voluntary control without the use of any instruments. Your major goal is to learn to lower muscle tension, anxiety level, and panic. Biofeedback training is well worth your time and effort, is something you will use in many situations and for years to come. Anxiety cannot be completely avoided, but it can be reduced. The problem with managing anxiety is reducing the anxiety to normal levels and then using the normal anxiety as stimulation to increase one's awareness.

Stress and anxiety put our body in a deficient state. Understanding your nutritional strengths and weaknesses is extremely important, but don't go out and buy a quantity of vitamins and "mega-dose." Mega-dosing won't do you any good, and will be a waste of good money. Locate an orthomolecular physician, therapist, or nutritionist, and get a complete evaluation.

Once you have established your nutritional needs, don't expect miracles. You've had the deficiencies for a while, and it takes time to rebuild your system. *There are no magic bullets.*

The amino acid therapy outlined in this book is used by orthomolecular physicians, therapists, and nutritional consultants.

If I suspect major amino acid deficiencies or multiple food allergies are the problem, I suggest my patients have a blood test. In addition to helping define nutrient status, an amino acid analysis can be useful in the detection and targeted treatment of a wide variety of disease states. This finding is possible because amino acids are involved in so many basic chemical reactions in the tissues. Amino acids make up the proteins found in every tissue of the body, playing a major role in nearly every chemical process that affects our physical and mental state. Some processes occur naturally, while others are synthesized with the help of enzymes and existing amino acids. Those amino acids not produced by the body must be supplied through dietary protein on a regular basis.

The body conducts a unique and very complicated series of chemical reactions in precisely controlled ways to give us what we have come to know as our health. There are over 5,000 reactions occurring each second in a cell. It is a wonder that we do not get sick more often. As busy as our brain is, it is the most under-nourished organ in the body.

Food allergy testing can provide you an easy and effective means of revealing foods that cause reactions. Researchers estimate that 60 percent of the U.S. population suffer from some reaction to foods that can cause or complicate a variety of health problems.

Depression

Most people think of their emotions as separate from their bodies and unconnected to the chemistry of their brain cells. However, depression, irritability, and anxiety all reflect functioning of the brain. When certain nutrients are not supplied to the brain, people experience an array of negative emotions, and tend to lose their coping ability in response to the stressful circumstances we confront each day of our lives.

Although the brain equals only two percent of our total body weight, 25 percent of our total metabolic activity takes place there. This is probably why the brain is so sensitive to nutritional deficiency. In fact, our need for proper brain function is so great that the body feeds the brain preferentially.

Nutrients can cause important changes in the chemical composition of substances in the brain, with corresponding changes in our feelings. Scientific studies demonstrate that by taking particular amino acids, depression, apathy, peevishness, and the desire to be left alone can be alleviated.

About one in five Americans has significant symptoms, more than 1.5 million are being treated for it, and approximately 30 million can expect to suffer from it at some point in their lives. Classic, full-blown depression has been described as "the loss of the capacity to enjoy life combined with a poverty of thought and movement." Depression can appear as grief, but manifests through a series of emotional states that can be so extreme that the outcome is suicide or total withdrawal.

Of course, a preoccupation with death or suicide is an obvious symptom, but often depression is not obvious because the person does not feel "sad." This is called "masked depression." Symptoms can involve changes in sleeping patterns, such as insomnia, early-morning waking, constant sleepiness, or changes in eating pattern (either overeating or loss of appetite). The person may be anxious or have excessive complaints about body functions and chronic pain, especially headaches, but also indigestion or constipation. Both hair and skin can feel dry and lose luster, while blood pressure has a tendency to be high. Symptoms usually include an inability to enjoy customary pleasures, and a concomitant loss of sex drive, loss of energy, extreme fatigue, difficulty concentrating and making decisions, irritability, and possibly temperamental outbursts.

With endogenous depression, symptoms include guilt, self-hate, feelings of worthlessness, apathy, crying spells, and a desire to be left alone. Women are more susceptible to depression than men—1 woman in 6 compared to 1 man in 12. There may be some connection to the female reproductive hormone cycles. Also, some diseases, such as hypothyroidism (underactive thyroid gland), produce depression, while others, such as arthritis or heart disease, commonly bring on a depressive reaction. Overall, not only can depression be a result of nutritional deficiency, but depression, in turn, further stresses the body. Without the proper nutritional attention, depression has a very deleterious effect on the general health.

If your moods and emotions are continuously clouded by the experiences of the past, you have to let go of the past. You must be free in the present to enjoy the present. Release the past, and let it rest in peace. Stay in the present and leave the depression in the past; it cannot come out with you *unless you bring it.* If your depression is caused by grief, multiple and complex problems can result. The aftermath of complex grief often leads to a constant fear of the illness suffered by the lost loved one. Grief and fear go hand-in-hand. Grief is as powerful as fear and can cause many years of suffering, if you do not deal with it properly. A behavior therapist who offers empathic understanding can help you put closure on this painful part of your life, and stay among the living.

Blood Flow and Panic Attacks

Studies indicate a difference in blood flow between the right and left sides of a specific brain area may cause panic attacks. Panic attacks seem to occur in the region of the brain believed to control emotions, in the limbic system, the amygdala, hippocampus, and caudate nucleus. The difference in blood flow between hemispheres is probably connected with differences in metabolic rate. Panic disorders could result when a hormone or neurotransmitter that normally regulates anxiety is missing or deficient.

Source: Daniel Carr, M.D. Massachusetts General Hospital.

VIII
Post Trauma
and Anxiety

Post Traumatic Stress Disorder (PTSD) affects one in twelve adults in the U.S. during their lifetime. Since 9-11 the figure has more than doubled. Traumatic events such as accidents, sexual assault, fire, floods, wartime experiences, major surgery, untimely loss of a loved one, or an act of terrorism such as 9-11, are all major triggers of PTSD. Post trauma can even affect those who watched the events of 9-11 on television. For four straight days the public was subjected to the events of that day, then a multitude of funerals that followed, and the grief suffered by those that lost loved ones. Now we are dealing with the fear and uncertainty of another attack, who knows when.

How does the brain process all of this information? What type of imprint will it leave? Acute stress disorder shares the following characteristics with PTSD: persistent symptoms of anxiety and panic, hyper arousal, fear of death, and total avoidance of stimuli associated with the traumatic experience. The brain imprint is part of the amygdala's processor—everything that you come in contact with, even before you are aware of what it is. The amygdala provides a preconscious reading of how the stimulus you come in contact with will affect you. It prepares you for the *fight-or-flight* response.

In *A User's Guide to the Brain* John Rately, M.D., states the amygdala's emotional tagging occurs simultaneously with memories that allow you to instantly judge and then react to an event. If the event of a situation is judged as dangerous, the amygdala sends signals for continued hyper arousal. Dr. Rately feels dopamine is a major key. Dopamine is abundant in the amygdala and is released in response to threatening events. This is why neurotransmitters are so vital to brain function. Dopamine strengthens the intense chemical firing of messages between neurons and allows neurons to communicate and identify a situation that tags them for future playback. The amino acid, Tyrosine, converts to dopamine in the brain and body.

Patients with acute stress disorder or post trauma will have a deficiency of neurotransmitters because of the constant hyper arousal. The brain will use all available neurotransmitters. All major neurotransmitters come from amino acids that must be supplied daily in specific amounts for the brain and body to be chemically balanced. A balanced neurotransmitter complex (SBNC) is the best approach to restore a stress-depleted brain. Post trauma symptoms can resurface even years after the event, such as Vietnam veterans have experienced.

According to Candace Pert, Ph.D., Pharmacologist and Researcher in amino acids, neurotransmitters, and neuropeptides, all of the emotions you feel during a traumatic event like 9-11 are felt by *every cell in your body.* When the amygdala releases playback messages, it can affect every part of your body. If you experienced trauma, find an empathetic behavior therapist that is not drug oriented to help you. Go over your experience, and as you do, you will notice your physical symptoms diminish; your symptoms decrease because you are desensitizing yourself. Learn relaxation therapy so you can breathe your way through it. Remember, deep breathing alone can change your brain chemistry. Use a combination of GABA, Glutamine, Tyrosine, L-Theanine, and SBNC to support your stressed brain and feed the amygdala and the rest of the limbic system. *Talk through your experiences. Each time you do, your symptoms will decrease and you will have more control.*

IX
The Self-Help Movement

The doctor of the future
will give no medicine
but will interest his patients
in the care of the human frame,
in diet, and in the cause and
prevention of disease.

Thomas A. Edison

The first time I saw a self-help magazine I was extremely happy—to say the least—that publishers were aware there was a need for this information. Then, month by month, more and more information on natural alternatives began to appear.

In 1976, I saw a report on L-tryptophan, the natural relaxant. I focused on "natural" and "relaxant" and realized there was an alternative to drugs and that many others were seeking the same thing. Searching for the new product at drugstores proved fruitless until, finally, one pharmacist suggested that a health food store should have L-tryptophan. It did. I slept better that night than I had in a long time. The tryptophan fed my brain that so desperately needed serotonin. Then, my search for information about amino acids began—and still goes on today.

The forerunners in research in the United States were Drs. Kenneth Pelletier and David Bresler, whose work in the field of psychosomatic pain and nutritional supplements opened many doors. In 1977, Dr. Pelletier released his best-selling book, *Mind as Healer, Mind as Slayer,* that sold a million copies its first year.

The book gives the reader the link between mind and body that is at the heart of health and disease. Dr. Pelletier gives a clear and concise picture of the power of the mind and how, as our stress level goes up, our painful, physical symptoms continue to occur until we cannot function. When I read this book in 1977, I learned the mind and body are one. They are inseparable. Our emotions are a bridge between the physical and mental systems that we experience. Dr. Pelletier introduces you to the new field of psychoneuroimmunology, or PNI, which brings together behavioral specialists, neurologists, and immunologists to explore the mind and body connection.

Dr. Bresler, past director of UCLA Pain Control Unit and a master practitioner of holistic health, was one of the first to use amino acids for pain and depression. In his book *Free Yourself from Pain*, Dr. Bresler covers the use of amino acids, especially studies using tryptophan and serotonin for chronic pain.

In 1980 Marilyn Ferguson published *The Aquarian Conspiracy,* which became a nonfiction top seller. This book talked about the personal and social transformation in the 80s. Under her section on "Healing Ourselves," she defines psychiatry as literally "doctoring the soul." It is unlikely that great doses of tranquilizing drugs can heal a fractured soul; rather, they interrupt the pattern of distress and conflict by altering the brain's disturbed chemistry.

It may take a bit more time for the medical profession, as a whole, to accept the concept of alternative therapies in general and non-drug treatment of stress and pain in particular, but as the information is brought to public attention, the change has begun. As patients realize there are alternatives to the usual rounds of toxic and addictive prescriptions to achieve freedom from pain, they will request natural products and alternative medicine. For example, acupuncture, massage, orthomolecular therapy, yoga, herbology, homeopathy, hypnosis, guided imagery, and biofeedback are now being sought out by a health-conscious public.

The integral approach is a new focus emerging within the health care community today, characterized by an integrated approach to the patient or individual. Rather than treating the individual parts, treatment centers around the *whole* person. Emphasis is placed on the psychological parts of the healing process, and the importance of maintaining health and wellness instead of the treatment of disease.

In the treatment of psychosomatic and psychosocial diseases of civilization, a variety of nonsomatic factors must be carefully examined. Such conditions as the inability to handle stress, a loss, or an adjustment effectively, problems in family or work environments, beliefs and expectations, having feelings of no control over your life, self-destructive habits, and a host of problems connected to human sexuality are all known to affect the onset of illness and the outcome of therapy. The enormous power of the mind is now being explored. A combination of mental, spiritual, and physical approaches can help to implement the body's intrinsic healing powers and ability for self-regulation in ways previously thought impossible. Further research may yield even more innovative techniques for creating and maintaining health.

Practitioners of integral medicine focus on the individual rather than a disease. They view the universal life force as a benevolent process that stimulates and supports human development. They view symptoms as a warning that something is wrong. These practitioners explore the meaning of illness through a therapeutic partnership in which patients and clinicians exchange information, advice, and support.

Integral medicine utilizes some aspects of holistic medicine, and it also uses "traditional" medicine. Integral medicine practitioners use individual combinations of both traditional and nontraditional approaches which place most of the responsibility with the patient in the treatment process. Using and integrating both the old and new methods of practice into the existing health care delivery system, offers the patient comprehensive care and help where he may not have been helped by symptomatic therapy. As a result, both the patients and their doctors are rediscovering the mutual trust and confidence that has traditionally been characteristic of the doctor-patient relationship.

The trend toward specialization is becoming more equilibrated by the search for an integrated understanding of the life process. Old rituals and new technologies are being brought together in unique and innovative ways. As a result, in the process both are altered, and the potential for total patient care is nearer to becoming a reality.

For example, for a patient who has injured his back *traditional* medicine would base treatment on drugs and surgery. *Alternative* medicine would focus on noninvasive alternative approaches. *Integral* medicine would draw from either or both and choose the best therapy for the individual needs of the patient. Further, traditional medicine believes that disease is caused primarily by physical factors. Alternative medicine emphasizes the mental, emotional, and social factors which are to blame. Integral medicine sees disease as a multifaceted process which results from an interaction of all these factors, each assuming different responsibilities.

This will be the medicine of the future and I thoroughly believe that the use of GABA is exciting and has a profound effect on the psychological as well as the physical feelings of the patient. In order to achieve the integral effect, other forms of therapy such as manipulation, nutritional counseling, therapeutic massage, biofeedback, homeopathy, hypnosis, and herbology—taking the best of two worlds—must not be overlooked, so that, in the end, the person who benefits is the *patient.*

Throughout this book I have discussed drastic changes in the way people view medicine, and their growing awareness of natural products such as GABA, tryptophan, DL-phenylalanine, glutamine, and other important nutrients available to replace painkillers and antidepressants. If not for the pioneers in the field, Dr. Kenneth Pelletier, David Bresler, Ph.D., Jeffrey Bland, Ph.D., Linus Pauling, Ph.D., Herbert Benson, M.D., Julian Whitaker, M.D., and Serafina Corsello, M.D., we might not be as far ahead at this point as we are now.

During the years 1975-76, any time the term "psychosomatic" was applied to a physical symptom, even physicians would turn away and avoid discussion of treatment for the patient. The strongest support for the validity of the term came from Dr. Pelletier's first book, *Mind as Healer, Mind as Slayer,* in which he emphatically defined psychosomatic medicine. At that point, 90 percent of the American public thought that a diagnosis of an illness as psychosomatic in nature meant that their pain was imaginary, that they were crazy, or that they had some type of emotional illness. Dr. Pelletier often refers to the "internist's bible," *Harrison's Principles of Internal Medicine,* which states that 50 to 80 percent of *all* disease is psychosomatic in nature. From this basis, he has defined psychosomatic illness as we know it today.

Psychosomatic illness does not mean that the patient has an emotional illness, nor that the pain is imaginary; the pain is real and the patient, indeed, suffers—even more so than with organic pathology. Pelletier emphatically went on record and named many illnesses being treated by all phases of medicine (ranging from peptic ulcers, migraines, ulcerated colitis, bronchial asthma, muscle spasms, and hay fever, to Raynaud's disease, hypertension, hyperthyroidism, rheumatoid arthritis, myositis, and edema), and he stated that these illnesses are stress-induced symptoms and that they are, in fact, psychosomatic in nature and have no pathology. Between 1975 and 1980 Drs. Pelletier, David Bresler, and Julian Whitaker began the campaign to inform and educate the public about the meaning of stress and anxiety-induced psychosomatic illness, and to teach them that not all psychosomatic illness requires traditional drugs.

The integral medicine approach was developed and implemented into a program for health care practitioners through UCLA Medical School. The founder and director of the Integral Medicine Program was Dr. Bresler. Other practitioners were Norman Shealy, M.D., Ph.D., Director of the Shealy Pain Clinic; Ronald Katz, M.D., Dennis Jaffe, Ph.D., Nancy Solomon, M.D., and Carl Simonton, M.D. In addition, pioneering clinicians and research scientists are now seriously investigating additional techniques that hold the promise of longer life and better health. As a result, therapeutic procedures once considered eccentric or esoteric are receiving increasing public acceptance and scientific validation.

In 1995 Bill Moyers' special on PBS, *Healing And The Mind*, presented the public with new breakthroughs in mind/body healing and medicine. Mr. Moyers' television series, followed by his book, is the most complete collection of provocative information available on mind/body medicine. This is the kind of information the American public is in search of, the natural alternative.

Most recently Caroline Myss, Ph.D., a medical intuitive and a pioneer in the field of energy medicine published *Anatomy of the Spirit* and *Why People Don't Heal*. Dr. Myss outlines how every illness corresponds to a pattern of psychological stresses, beliefs, and attitudes that influence corresponding areas of the body. Her research follows the same philosophy as Dr. Kenneth Pelletier's regarding the relationship between mental stress and physical symptoms.

In her book *Molecules of Emotion* Candace Pert states, "Information molecules are peptides and receptors. They are the biochemicals of emotions. These molecules are found in parts of the brain that mediate our emotions. They control the opening and closing of blood vessels in your face. They allow the systems in the body to talk to each other. They carry messages within the brain and from the brain to the body. *The mind and body are one; they cannot be separated."*

X
Self-Help
Information

The following exercise will help you relax and reduce your anxiety and stress. Deep breathing exercises will help you get through the anxious times and not become tense. The exercises will also correct shallow breathing. Always breath in through your nose and out through your mouth. Release the air slowly, this will help reduce muscle tension. You can use this exercise in your car, at work, or at home. The more you practice, the faster you will feel the benefits. Let yourself go to your own corner of the world, a place where you feel safe, warm, and relaxed. Take slow, deep breaths, and scan your body for tension; then release it by blowing out gently. Do not think about inhaling. Just let the air come in naturally, let your shoulders drop, and your stomach muscles relax. Focus only on your own corner of the world, and allow yourself to let go and relax. Remember, deep breathing can change the chemistry of the brain and release neurotransmitters.

Relaxation Exercise

My mind is still . . .
If I have any thoughts or worries,
I will let them float away . . .
I am at peace . . .
I will breathe gently and deeply and just relax . . .
My body is resting and healing . . .

I am calm . . .
I am safe and at peace . . .
I will relax and let my fear drift away . . .
I am at peace . . .
I am healing . . .
My mind and body are one.

How to Stop P.A.s
(Panic Attacks)

1. If you feel frightened, bewildered, unreal, or unsteady, *know* that these feelings are nothing more than an *exaggeration* of the normal bodily reactions to stress.

2. The fact that you have these sensations does not mean you are sick. These feelings are just unpleasant and frightening, not dangerous. Nothing worse will happen to you.

3. Let your feelings come. They've been in charge of you. You've been pumping them up and making them more acute. Stop pumping. Don't run away from panic. When you feel the panic mount, take a deep breath and as you breathe out, blow it out, let it go. Stay there almost as if you were floating in space. Don't fight the feeling of panic. Accept it. The more you fight panic, the stronger the feelings become.

4. Try to make yourself as comfortable as possible without trying to escape. If you're on a street, lean against a post or a wall. If you're in a department store, find a quiet corner. If you're in a grocery store, tell the salesperson you don't feel well and want to sit for a while. Do not jump into your car and go home in fear.

5. Stop adding to your panic with frightening thoughts about what is happening and where it might lead. Don't indulge in self-pity and think, "Why can't I be like other people? Why do I have to go through all this?" Just accept what is happening to you. If you do this, what you fear most will not happen.

6. Think about what is really happening to your body at this moment. Do not think, "Something terrible is going to happen. I must get out." Repeat to yourself, "I will not fall, faint, die, or lose control." Nothing is going to happen!

7. Now, wait and give the fear time to pass. Do not run away. Others have conquered the fear, and so will you. Notice that as you stop thinking about your fear, the fear will start to fade away by itself.

8. This is your opportunity to practice. Think of it that way. Even if you feel isolated in space, soon that will pass. Sometime soon you will be able to go through the panic and say, "I did it! I am in control, not the fear." Think about the progress you have already made. If you have a tendency to hyperventilate, focus on your breathing. Your breathing should be *slow and deep*. You should breathe in through your nose and out through your mouth. This stops the gasping that causes hyperventilation. Your healing has begun and will continue.

9. Try to distract yourself from what is going on inside you. Look at your surroundings. See the other people on the street, in the bus. They are with you, not against you.

10. When the panic subsides, let your body go loose, take a deep breath, and go on with your day. Remember, each time you cope with a panic attack, you reduce your fear.

How to Take a Pill or Capsule
(According to the American Medical Association)

The right way to make the medicine go down depends on whether it is a tablet or a capsule. You won't have to worry about aspirin sticking to the roof of your mouth, or vitamins lodging in your throat, if you follow this simple procedure.

Tablet   With a full glass of water at hand, place the pill on your tongue, tilt your head back, and take a swallow of water.

Capsule   The procedure is similar for a capsule, except that you should tilt your head or upper body *forward*. Since capsules are lighter than water, they will float to the back of your mouth and go down smoothly.

Symptoms of Hyperventilation /Hysteria

Headache

Dizziness

Shortness of breath

Hands numb or tingling

Dry mouth

Feeling unsteady

Feeling faint

Feeling nauseated

Having little stamina and tiring easily

Pain in the chest

Dizziness while lying down or sitting

Feet numb or tingling

Trouble thinking clearly

Feeling light headed

Trembling hands

Feeling of tightness in the chest

Blurred vision

Passing out, unconscious

Feeling a lump in the throat

Ringing or whistling in the ears

Feeling "far away"

Difficulty talking

Cold, pale hands

Feeling of breathing "too much"

Feeling excited for no reason

Waking up at night short of breath

Face numb or tingling

Hands tight and hard to open

Feeling that everything is unreal

Crying for no good reason

Tongue numb or tingling

Seeing double

Laughing for no good reason

Source: *Hyperventilation and Hysteria,* by Thomas P. Lowry, M.D.

Hyperventilation

Hyperventilation is an insidious condition, gradually developing over a period of years, in which the victim unconsciously over breathes, releasing too much carbon dioxide from his body. This remarkably prevalent disorder affects, to some extent, a fifth of all adults. Hyperventilation tends to be unnerving, since it can be a marvelously mimic such diverse disorders as stroke, epilepsy, multiple sclerosis, and heart disease. By far, the most common cause of dizziness, breathlessness, and numbness around the lips or in the limbs in younger people is hyperventilation. Hyperventilation can also produce nausea, tremulousness, cold hands and feet, palpitations, and chest pain—the latter often misdiagnosed as a coronary when the pain is accompanied by alarming changes in the electrocardiogram.

The psychogenic causes of hyperventilation are fear, anger, anxiety, panic, grief, and hysteria. Hyperventilation syndrome can completely control the body chemistry—it's a perfect example of how the mind changes the body, and how bodily changes can produce emotional and psychological sensations.

Most chronic hyperventilators are unaware of their over breathing. A physician is seldom able to detect this abnormal breathing pattern unless he provokes its characteristic symptoms by having the patient deliberately hyperventilate.

How are hyperventilators treated? A simple explanation of the disorder (along with the strong reassurance that it does not represent some life-threatening disease of the heart, lungs, or brain) and instructions on how to breathe properly usually work wonders. Also, careful instruction in such preventive maneuvers as prolonged breath-holding, or breathing carbon dioxide-rich expired air through a paper bag.

If these techniques do not prevent further attacks, another approach can be tried—biofeedback and self hypnosis training. I hyperventilated at one time during my phobic year and found this to be the most effective. Those who are mouth breathers have a tendency to hyperventilate. Your breathing should be slow and deep. Breathe in through your nose and out through your mouth. This stops the gasping that causes hyperventilation.

Stress-Anxiety Reactions

Within 24 to 48 hours after anxiety, stress, anger, or an emotional upset reaction, major physical symptoms often occur. The body requires more amino acids and nutrients. The following physical symptoms can occur.

Headaches	Increased sweating
Face/body aches	Increased anxiety
Neck and back pain	Jaw clenching
Muscle spasms	Skin eruption/acne
Trigger points	Elevated blood pressure
Sleep loss	Bladder infections
Indigestion	Ulcers
Upset stomach	Constipation
Diarrhea	Increased pain
Pounding heart	Changes in sexual interest

The three types of stress include emotional, chemical, and physical. Physiological changes in different organs can lead to weakening of the organ and the immune system. If the prolonged anxiety or stress continues, a disease state can follow. Replenishing your neurotransmitters relieves emotional, chemical, and physical symptoms, and fortifies the body.

Anxiety and Depression Medication Withdrawal Symptoms

Weight loss
Chills
Hiccups
Low-back pain
Muscle twitching
Muscle weakness
Tremors
Weakness
Apathy
Craving for the medication
Delirium
Depression
Dizziness
Fatigue
Insomnia
Irritability
Loss of appetite
Nightmare
Panic
Anger
Rage
Crawling sensations on the skin
Seizures
Gooseflesh
Rashes
Incontinence
Stomachaches
Intestinal cramps
Nausea and vomiting
Diarrhea
Constipation
Yawning
Bad taste in mouth

Aching in the ears
Runny nose
Smelling unpleasant odors
Watery eyes
Uncontrolled blinking
Rapid movement of the eyes
Dilated pupils
Double vision
Headaches
Muscle contraction headaches
Increased anxiety
Panic or anxiety attacks
Agoraphobia
Flu-like symptoms
Hyperactivity
Hallucinations
Confusion
Sweating
Palpitations
Slow or rapid pulse
Tight chest
Abdominal pain
Restlessness
Increased sensitivity to noise,
    light, touch, or smell
Change in sexual interest
Impotence
Pains in the shoulder, neck,
    jaw, or face
Chronic pain
Jitteriness
Shaking

The length of withdrawal symptoms varies from individual to individual. Variables include length of time the drug was taken, the age of the person, the stress level, and the state of nutrition. Increased anxiety after a drug has been stopped is not uncommon, and can be lead to rebound anxiety. Symptoms diminish as the level of neurotransmitters are produced and replenished. The key lies in following an orthomolecular program and giving the body and mind time to heal.

Anxiety/Magnesium Connection

Magnesium deficiency symptoms:

Anxiety
Panic attacks
Mitral valve prolapse
Hypertension
Chronic pain
Back and neck pain
Muscle spasms
Migraines
Fibromyalgia
Spastic symptoms
Chronic bronchitis
Dizziness
Confusion
Depression
Noise and light sensitivity
Ringing in the ears
Irritable bowel syndrome
Heart disease
Cardiac arrhythmias
Atherosclerosis
Cold hands and feet
TIAs (Transient Ischemic
    Attacks—strokes)
Constipation
Fatigue
Diabetes
Hypoglycemia
Asthma
Seizures
Kidney stones
PMS syndrome
Menstrual cramps
Osteoporosis

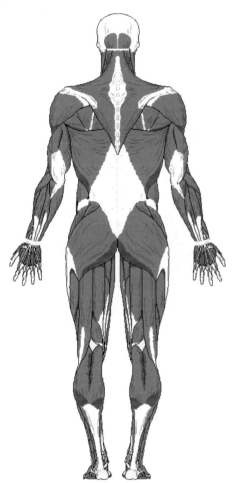

Magnesium is the *number one stress* mineral, and plays an important role in the control of anxiety. Magnesium is a *cofactor* for all amino acids. To reduce anxiety, use magnesium in the form of magnesium chloride (Mag Link capsules or Mag Chlor 85 liquid). If you have added GABA and other amino acids to your program and still feel anxious, add magnesium chloride twice to three times daily. Your anxiety symptoms will start to diminish.

Cycle of Feelings

Anxiety is the fear of hurt or loss, nagging stress.

Hurt, or *loss,* leads to anger, anxiety, uncertainty.

Anger held in leads to guilt, depression, frustration.

Guilt, unexpressed, leads to depression.

Fear which is not confronted or understood becomes avoidance.

Avoidance of unresolved feelings leads to phobias.

Phobias lead to a constant control by overwhelming fear.

Fear leads to pain, physical and emotional.

Pain leads to fear, rational and irrational.

Uncertainty is nagging stress.

Repression is forcing a thought to the subconscious.

Frustration is loss of objectivity.

Dependency is need for a specific effect.

Resentment is mixed emotions, unsorted.

Depersonalization is loss of identity.

Denial is refusal to admit reality.

Grief is the psychological and physical trauma of loss.

Sadness is the sense of loss, and abnormal daily functioning.

XI
Nutritional Medicine

Amino Acids

*D**LPA (DL-phenylalanine),* an essential amino acid, helps control depression and chronic pain. Studies since 1972 at John Hopkins University School of Medicine demonstrate DLPA is particularly beneficial in cases of endogenous depression. Endogenous depression is characterized by a decrease in energy and interest, feelings of worthlessness, and a pervasive sense of helplessness to control the course of a person's life. Significant improvement has been achieved with people suffering from several types of depression such as grief, age-related depression, mania, schizophrenia, and post-amphetamine depression.

In his book, *DLPA to End Chronic Pain and Depression,* Arnold Fox, M.D., describes the three separate antidepressant effects of DLPA in the body and brain. The first is increased production of PEA (phenylethylamine), a neurotransmitter-type substance that acts as a natural stimulant in the brain function. The second action of DLPA as an antidepressant is its ability to inhibit enzymes which breakdown the endorphin hormone. Endorphins are morphine-like substances produced by the body. Endorphins have a specific action in the brain, critical to mood regulation. The third major function of DLPA's antidepressants effects is the creation of norepinephrine. These three biochemical actions are not isolated, but rather create a synergistic overlap accounting for the effective result of DLPA in the treatment of depression.

DLPA is converted to the neurotransmitter norepinephrine in the brain. A deficiency of norepinephrine causes depression. Norepinephrine and PEA are both natural stimulants. In 1979 published reports found DLPA to be equally as effective as the tricyclic drug, Imipramine, one of the top three prescribed antidepressants in the U.S. The reports were the results of controlled double-blind studies of patients suffering long-term depression.

DLPA is not a drug, and is an essential amino acid that has no adverse side effects and is not habit-forming. DLPA is an effective safe antidepressant that can be taken on a regular basis. DLPA has also been shown to be effective for alleviating P.M.S. and the swelling of arthritis and chronic pain.

The recommended dose is 750 mg with breakfast, lunch, and dinner. DLPA should be taken with meals or within one hour of completing a meal. DLPA is nontoxic and non-addictive. Chronic low-back and neck pain responds to DLPA. *Do not use L-Tyrosine, L-Phenylalanine, or DLPA if you are taking MAO or tricyclic antidepressants.*

L-Tyrosine helps in overcoming depression, improving memory, increasing mental alertness, relieving Obsessive Compulsive Disorder (OCD), and depression. Of particular interest is the research linking L-tyrosine deficiency to the increased craving of cocaine and alcohol.

The body needs L-tyrosine to build many complex structural proteins and enzymes, but the recent clinical research has centered on the simpler compounds used by the body to transmit nerve impulses and to determine one's mental mood and alertness. These compounds are called neurotransmitters, and they are readily formed in the body by minor alteration of the L-tyrosine molecule. Research suggests that, very likely deficiencies of L-tyrosine can impair the body's ability to produce the proper balance of these neurotransmitters.

The best food sources of L-tyrosine are meats, eggs, and dairy products. Clinical researchers prefer to use L-tyrosine supplements, rather than rely on whole foods, because it is difficult to obtain needed amounts in normal diets. L-tyrosine (or its precursor, L-phenylalanine) is used by the body to produce several compounds important to nerve transmission.

Two compounds, epinephrine and norepinephrine, have wide-ranging activities that affect brain and nerve cells. Both compounds are produced in nerve cells, as well as in the adrenal medulla where they can be stored. A third compound produced from L-tyrosine, dopamine, affects nerve tracts in the brain, and also functions in the production of the other two.

Neurotransmitters control impulse transmission between nerve cells, allowing the cells to talk to each other. Nerve terminals in the hypothalamus secrete epinephrine. Sympathetic nerve (*fight-or-flight response*) endings release norepinephrine and, thus, affect the firing of the cells.

These neurotransmitters are responsible for an elevated and positive mood, alertness, and concentration. Medical researchers in the past have relied on increasing the brain and nerve levels of norepinephrine by using drugs such as phenylpropanolamine and amphetamines. Drugs cause the release of norepinephrine, block its return to storage, or slow the destruction of L-tyrosine. However, such artificial manipulation often leads to depletion of the neurotransmitter and the aggravation of the original problem. The natural solution is to normalize brain and nerve levels of norepinephrine by providing adequate levels of the amino acids.

Clinical studies demonstrate L-tyrosine controls medication-resistant depression. If taken properly, L-tyrosine can benefit those suffering from chronic depression. Our protocol at the Pain & Stress Center is 850 mg every morning and evening. If you are 100 pounds or less, tyrosine (500 mg twice daily) gives you the lift you need. Make sure you take 25 mg of B6 daily to activate the tyrosine. L-tyrosine is now used in many drug rehabilitation programs to stop the craving of cocaine. *Caution: Do not use L-Tyrosine, L-Phenylalanine, or DLPA if you are taking MAO, tricyclic or SSRI antidepressants, or if you have a history or a melanoma. Pregnant or lactating women should consult a health care professional.*

L-Glutamine is an inhibitory neurotransmitter and the precursor for GABA, the anti-anxiety amino acid. Glutamine's major function is memory, concentration, and inhibition. Scientific research has disclosed glutamine has multiple benefits in body function. Glutamine has a direct link to the smooth functioning of the musculoskeletal system and aids in muscle development after a long illness causing muscle wasting. Glutamine transports waste ammonia from peripheral organs, especially the muscles, kidneys, gut, and brain, to the liver, where the detoxification process occurs. In the kidney, ammonia is excreted via the urine. Glutamine helps the brain dispose of waste ammonia as well as other toxic substances. Glutamine helps strengthen the immune system, and enhances and supports pancreatic growth. Glutamine is released into the blood or diffuses into neurons where the neurotransmitters glutamate and GABA form from glutamine.

For many years, glutamine was considered a nonessential amino acid, but research over the past several years has brought forth a wave of important new information that changed this view. In the 1980s, glutamine was reestablished as a conditionally-essential amino acid. Under normal circumstances, the body can make adequate amounts of the amino acid. Under prolonged stress, anxiety, panic, trauma, or illness, the body cannot produce enough and the body requires glutamine supplements. New research demonstrates up to one-third of the amino acids released during times of stress and anxiety is in the form of glutamine. Taking glutamine with balanced amino acids essentially prevents muscle breakdown (atrophy). This amazing amino acid, along with GABA and glycine, is rapidly becoming the most important therapeutic amino acid of the twenty-first century.

The amino acid trio of glutamine, GABA, glycine and B6, the cofactor, make up the major inhibitory neurotransmitters in the brain. Glutamine is found in the nerves of the hippocampus, the memory center of the brain, in the cranial nerves, and in many other areas of the brain. These three amino acids work together and are inhibitory neurotransmitters, the chemical language of the brain.

Glutamine studies reported that children and adults demonstrating symptoms of A.D.D. had an increase in IQ after taking glutamine in combination with ginkgo and B6. Research done by Dr. Roger Williams at the University of Texas, Clayton Foundation, revealed children and adults classified A.D.H.D. had a marked improvement when taking 500 to 1,000 mg of glutamine daily. Dosage depends on age and weight.

GABA and glutamine are *not only* found in the brain but in the receptor sites throughout the body. Amino acids can and do change mind, mood, memory, and behavior.

For alcohol craving, Dr. Roger Williams, pioneer in glutamine research, found that 3,000 to 4,000 milligrams of glutamine daily stops the craving for alcohol and decreases the craving for sweets. Since glutamine is tasteless and mixes with water or any liquid, it is easy to take. Our patients also reported a lift from fatigue, both mental and physical. One alcoholic stopped drinking when glutamine was administered daily. Two years later the patient was still free from the craving for alcohol. He has maintained a nutritional support program. Glutamine was given to one group of alcoholics and placebos to the other. The group taking at least three thousand milligrams of glutamine daily were free of alcohol craving.

Glutamine is converted to energy by the brain and is the brain's main fuel. Glutamine is converted to GABA with the help of magnesium. Without continued high energy in the brain, the rest of the mind and body will NOT function properly. The brain requires tremendous quantities of glucose and oxygen in order to function correctly. This is supplied via the bloodstream to ensure the brain receives the energy it needs.

The main nutrient needed for intestinal repair is glutamine. Leaky gut syndrome is seen more often today due to the increased use of anti-inflammatory medications such as Lodeine, Oruvail, Motrin, Advil, Ibuprofen, Dolobid, Anaprox, Orudis, Naprosyn, etc. Leaky gut syndrome makes the intestines more permeable and allows in substances and foods which normally do not pass into the circulation. Food allergies can result, causing more discomfort and pain. But glutamine helps the gut heal and makes the intestines less permeable. Japanese researchers established glutamine helps stomach ulcers heal. For leaky gut, use Glutamine 1000 powder, 2,000 mg twice to three times daily, divided.

In cancer patients glutamine enhances the effectiveness of chemotherapy and radiation treatments while reducing the toxicity and damage to the body. Dosages vary in amounts, but a rule of thumb is 0.5 gram /kilogram /day. Patients had decreased systemic infections (sepsis), less weight loss, decreased mortality, and increased healing rates of radiated intestines. For best results, glutamine should be taken prior to treatment and continued throughout therapy.

Unfortunately, foods are not a good source of glutamine. The foods highest in glutamine include meat, chicken, and eggs, but in the RAW form. Cooking or heat inactivates glutamine, so your best source is in supplement form.

Glutamine is truly an amazing amino acid with multiple benefits, and, with continued research, other important factors will be found that will improve our quality of life.

Taurine is a naturally-occurring amino acid that is highly concentrated in animal and fish proteins. The body manufactures taurine from methionine or cysteine in the liver when B6 is present. Taurine is found in appreciable amounts in excitable tissue such as the heart, skeletal muscle, eye, and the central nervous system, including the brain. Taurine is the most plentiful amino acid in the developing brain and the second most abundant in the brain after glutamic acid. No wonder disturbances in taurine metabolism are seen in problems as diverse as heart disease and epilepsy.

Taurine protects and stabilizes the brain's fragile membranes and acts as a neurotransmitter. Taurine seems to be closely related in its structure and metabolism to other neurotransmitters such as glycine and GABA. Taurine, like GABA, is inhibitory. Taurine, or a modified taurine, may someday supersede synthetic tranquilizers. Women require more taurine than men since estradiol is found to inhibit its synthesis in the liver. Some studies found significantly decreased levels of taurine in depressed patients. This has been confirmed with amino acid analysis.

Taurine has a potent anticonvulsant action. Most studies find taurine is diminished in epileptic and seizure patients. Taurine intakes between 200 and 1,500 mg per day helps with epileptic seizures. However, higher doses of taurine may be required. Taurine assists people with tics or other spastic conditions.

Taurine improves fat metabolism in the liver, seems to play a role with cholesterol, and helps prevent the formation of gall stones. Taurine helps conserve potassium and calcium in the heart muscle, thereby helping the heart to function more efficiently. As with most nutrients, the body's need for taurine increases whenever an individual is under stress.

Glycine is the simplest nonessential amino acid. It resembles glucose (blood sugar) and glycogen (liver starch). Glycine is sweet to taste and can be used as a sweetener. It can mask bitterness and saltiness. Pure glycine dissolves easily in liquids. Glycine is probably the third major inhibitory neurotransmitter in the brain. Glycine readily passes the blood-brain barrier.

Although glycine is not an essential amino acid, it is an essential intermediate in the metabolism of proteins, peptides, and bile salts. Glycine, taurine, and GABA are the major inhibitory neurotransmitters in the brain and central nervous system (C.N.S.). Glycine is a very nontoxic amino acid. Even with doses up to 30 grams, glycine has not produced side effects.

Glycine is involved with convulsions and retinal function. Glycine taken orally increases the urinary excretion of uric acid, and is possibly useful in preventing gout.

Glycine, like taurine, seems to be important in reducing the symptoms of epilepsy and spasticity. In addition, glycine alleviates the toxic effects of substances such as phenol, benzoic acid, and lead. Glycine may be used to reduce aggression, since glycine can have a sedative effect. In one study, glycine in large doses ended an acute manic episode within one hour. Glycine helps trigger brain cells to fire electrical charges that speed learning.

Lysine, an essential amino acid, is found in large quantities in muscle tissue. B6 is important for increasing the absorption of lysine. B6 is the lysine cofactor. Stress and anxiety, as with all emotions, have a negative effect on our emotional skin. Within 24 to 48 hours after an emotional outpouring or stress reaction, the skin reflects it. Cold sores, facial and body blisters, and herpes are the most prevalent. Genital herpes is also a response to stress reactions. Lysine is effective in the treatment of herpes and other skin problems. Clinical studies demonstrated lysine effective in reducing the severity of herpes and cold sore attacks, with accelerated healing time. Non active stages require 1000 mg daily. During acute attacks, increase the lysine to 2,000 to 3,000 mg per day. Other beneficial nutrients include Ester C with bioflavonoids, 2,000 to 3,000 mg daily, divided; and zinc picolinate, 30 mg daily. A lysine cream available for topical use helps relieve pain. In reduced doses, lysine is safe for children.

Methionine is an essential sulfur amino acid that performs three major roles in the body. Methionine is a methyl donor, sulfur donor, and a precursor of synthesis of other sulfur amino acids. The interactions of Vitamin B12, folate, magnesium, and B6, with methionine play a very important part in normal methionine metabolism. Methionine studies support methionine's antidepressant properties. Some researchers report methionine is as effective as two popular antidepressants, clomipramine and amitriptyline (Elavil).

Patients with high histamine levels found methionine extremely helpful in lowering the histamine and elevating depressed moods, in some cases more effectively than MAO inhibitors. Those patients had a marked improvement presented with symptoms of asthma, chronic pain syndrome, fibromyalgia, allergies, depression, and high cholesterol. Take 1,000 to 2,000 mg methionine with timed-release B6 and magnesium.

GABA 750. GABA (Gamma Amino Butyric Acid) is a major inhibitory neurotransmitter. Dr. Candace Pert, Pharmacologist, discovered through her research that there are GABA receptors sites throughout the body and brain. Stress and anxiety deplete GABA levels in the brain and body. GABA helps cool the brain. Amino acid deficiencies occur when we experience long periods of stress, anxiety, depression, or pain. Stress affects the limbic system, the feelings part of the brain, and uses available neurotransmitters such as GABA. When the brain is bombarded by anxiety signals, you become anxious, tense, and feel out of control. GABA has a natural calming effect. GABA 750 was described by Dr. Julian Whitaker in *Health & Healing*, March 1994. Recommended dosage is ½ capsule dissolved in water or under the tongue, three times daily if under 125 pounds. If over 125 pounds, dissolve one capsule in water or under your tongue, three times daily. Recently, **GABA 375** became available. You can use this instead of ½ capsule. It is pure pharmaceutical grade GABA in capsule form. As with the GABA 750, the capsule should be opened and dissolved in water.

5-HTP, or 5-Hydroxytryptophan, is the precursor to serotonin in the brain and, as a supplement derives from the griffonia seed. Serotonin is a calming neuro-nutrient and helps reduce anxiety, anger, and aggression while enhancing sleep when taken at bedtime. 5-HTP is available in 50 mg capsules or in 10 mg combination product known as HTP10. Always use pharmaceutical-grade aminos. Use 50 mg of 5-HTP if you weigh over 50 pounds. *CAUTION: Do not take 5-HTP if you are taking SSRI (Selective Serotonin Reuptake Inhibitors) or MAO inhibitors.*

L-Theanine is a new amino acid that derives from green tea leaves that has recently come to the forefront. Studies demonstrate

L-Theanine increases alpha brain waves (like deep meditation) while reducing muscle tension, stress and anxiety. Another study in the *Journal of Food Science and Technology* show that L-Theanine releases neurotransmitters such as dopamine and serotonin. Theanine appears to play a role in the formation of GABA. Other clinical research demonstrates that theanine creates a sense of well-being, calm, and relaxation plus other helpful properties. You can use Theanine to assist when you are coming off medications when other amino acids are prohibited. Theanine helps you remain calm and relaxed, and is excellent to use during and after your withdrawal period. My book, *Break Your Prescribed Addiction* offers help coming off tranquilizers, antidepressants, and more. For more information L-Theanine, read my book, *Theanine, The Relaxation Amino Acid.*

Important Notice

If you are taking prescriptions drugs,
DO NOT JUST STOP TAKING THEM!
Withdrawal reactions can occur. Consult your physician or a qualified health care professional for help.

Special Amino Acids Formulations

Anxiety Control 24. AC 24, a patented amino acid support formula, combines amino acids, herbs, minerals, and essential cofactors to help relax the anxious or stressed mind and body. After many years of research I formulated Anxiety Control. This formula contains the major inhibitory neurotransmitters in the brain, which are GABA, glycine, and glutamine. Neurotransmitters are the chemical language of the brain. B6 is the major cofactor for activation of amino acids in the body. The herbs Passion Flower and Primula Officinalis support an overstressed body and calm the central nervous system naturally. Anxiety Control 24 can be used all day, or at night, to feed the brain deficiencies created in today's stressful lifestyles. Anxious or overly active teens and children can use this product safely. Recommended dosage for anyone over 100 pounds, is up to 4 daily.

S.B.N.C. (Super Balanced Neurotransmitter Complex) Neurotransmitters assist in effective brain communication. S.B.N.C. provides your brain the needed nutrients to enhance maximum brain function. An unbalanced diet, anxiety, and stress, plus other factors, can contribute to disturbances in amino acid metabolism. Many people have undetected impairments of their biochemistry that can either cause or complicate their health condition. Amino acids are intimately involved in metabolic regulation, and are proving very useful as therapeutic agents that reverse the biochemical impairments related to amino acid metabolism. Amino acid therapy can be instrumental in correcting or reducing stress and anxiety, chronic fatigue, food and chemical intolerances, frequent headaches, recurrent infections, mental and emotional disturbances, hyperactivity, learning disabilities, neurological disorders, drug cravings, and eating disorders. Take S.B.N.C. with some fruit juice to facilitate the rapid uptake of the amino acids. Recommended dosage is 1 or 2 capsules, twice daily.

Brain Link is an amino acid complex that creates the neurotransmitter link for enhanced brain function. Brain Link is a total formula for daily use, and can be used in conjunction with all other supplements. I formulated Brain Link, the most complete neurotransmitter formula available on the market today. Brain Link is perfect for all ages, 1 to 100. Recommended dosage is by weight. Children up to 75 pounds take two scoops, those 75–120 pounds take four scoops, and others over 120 pounds take six scoops daily in divided doses.

Pain Control is a special combination of amino acids and anti-inflammatory herbs that have special pain-reducing properties.

This combination has been used at the Pain & Stress Center in our pain program with excellent success. Pain Control is excellent for stress-induced pain and tension. Pain Control contains DLPA, Boswellia, GABA, Ashwagandha, and B6. For maintenance use one to two capsules every four to six hours as needed, up to eight daily. (*NOTE: Do not take MAO or tricyclic anti-depressants with DL-phenylalanine.*)

Mood Sync is a special combination of 5-HTP, L-Tyrosine, GABA, glutamine, taurine, and B6. This combination reduces stress, and anxiety while lifting your mood. Mood Sync provides the proper amino acids to address and restore brain imbalances caused by stress, depression, anger, aggression, mood swings, and P.M.S. Mood Sync can be taken during the day, or at bedtime. Usual dosage is one to two capsules, two to three times daily. *Caution: Do not use Mood Sync if you are taking MAO, SSRI or tricyclic antidepressants, or if you have a history of melanoma.*

HTP10 is a combination of 5-HTP (10 mg) with GABA, glycine, glutamine, lysine, taurine, magnesium, Vitamins B6 and C, and Alpha KG. HTP10 can be used by children or smaller adults; doses greater than 10 mg of 5-HTP can cause drowsiness or sleepiness in some patients. *CAUTION: Do not take 5-HTP if you are taking SSRI (Selective Serotonin Reuptake Inhibitors), MAO inhibitors, or tricyclic antidepressants .*

L–T is a combination of L-Theanine, GABA, and Glutamine. L-Theanine is the relaxation amino acid that derives from green tea leaves. L–T calms the brain without drowsiness or a dull feeling. Dosage: one to two capsules, three to four times daily, divided to a maximum of eight.

Sleep Link is a special combination sleep formula that contains melatonin, L-Theanine, 5-HTP, GABA, Passion Flower, Ashwagandha, and Glutamine. Sleep Link helps you obtain the needed sleep your brain and body require for healing and repairs. Sleep disturbances occur when brain neurotransmitters become out of balance due to chronic anxiety or stress or depression. Sleep

Link helps replenish your neurotransmitter levels so your sleep disturbances resolve. The melatonin combined with 5-HTP in Sleep Link helps balance your circadian rhythm. Dosage: Use one or two Sleep Link, 30 minutes before bedtime. For a super bedtime cocktail, combine two Sleep Link with Mag Chlor 85. Use 15 to 25 drops of Mag Chlor 85 in water or juice.

B AND C—The Water Soluble Vitamins

Vitamin B is actually a "complex" of several vitamins including B1–thiamine, B2–riboflavin, B3–niacin (niacinamide), B6–pyridoxine, B12–cyanocobalamin, pantothenic acid (calcium pantothenate), biotin, PABA (paraaminobenzoic acid), folic acid, choline, and inositol. All the B vitamins are water soluble and are excreted via the kidneys in the urine. They are not stored in the body and, therefore, must be supplied in sufficient amounts at all times—especially when the body is under stress of any kind.

Even though the B vitamins are supplied in the diet in quantities to support normal health, this supply can be inadequate under stress unless the Bs are supplied in good amounts. *Stress* is anything causing extra tension—emotional and/or physical—on the body; for example: drugs, alcohol, chemicals, excessive fatigue, noise, infections, emotional turmoil, and anxiety. Recall that alcohol is a source of energy (calories) in the body; alcohol is definitely a carbohydrate and is broken down to sugar in the body. The B vitamins are required in the burning of alcohol in the body. If large amounts of carbohydrates are consumed, the individual should also increase his daily intake of the B vitamins.

As a complex, the B vitamins play a significant role in alleviating depression and in relieving the anxiety and restlessness that often accompany it, perhaps, partially due to the effect of the B vitamins on lactic acid. Certain metabolic processes and exercise produce the formation of lactic acid when there is inadequate B vitamins or oxygen. If you exercise strenuously without gradually building up, lactic acid accumulates in your muscles. Excessive lactic acid can produce anxiety and painful muscle spasms.

The first clinical effects of inadequate B vitamins are insomnia, mood changes, decreased immune function, impaired drug metabolism, and sugar cravings.

Vitamin B6 (Pyridoxine) plays a major role in regulating your moods and is often indicated in the cause and treatment of depression. B6 might better be termed the Enabler vitamin. Vitamin B6 literally controls all the amino acid metabolism and transformations in your body. The body requires B6 for the proper functioning of over 60 metabolic and enzymatic processes in the body. Without adequate B6, the amino acids are not of much value to you. B6 also controls amino acid absorption from your gastrointestinal tract. B6 is involved in carbohydrate and fat metabolism, as well as the formation of red blood cells and antibodies.

The average American diet tends to be high in protein and fat. Such a diet causes an increased requirement of B6. Stress, alcohol consumption, tobacco, birth control pills, pregnancy, and medications further deplete the levels of B6.

B6 is available in 150 mg timed-release capsules released over 9 to 10 hours.

Pyridoxal 5' Phosphate (P5'P) is the biological form of B6, reportedly ten times more potent then B6. Taking P5'P is another way to ensure adequate intake of B6 without worrying about taking too much. P5'P does not have any side effects and can be taken by both children and adults. A deficiency of P5'P causes increased excretion of most amino acids.

Ester C Polyascorbate—Vitamin C. In attempting to achieve optimum nutrition, the major obstacle preventing efficient absorption of Vitamin C is *acid rejection syndrome.* This rejection occurs when acidic Vitamin C (ascorbic acid) enters the alkaline environment of the lower digestive tract, which is where most of the Vitamin C is absorbed. This acidic rejection by the duodenum and the small and large intestines causes inflamed tissue, flatulence, diarrhea, and discomfort, resulting in minimal absorption. The irritation often goes undetected because of the limited number of sensory nerves in the digestive tract.

Even so-called buffered Vitamin C, timed-released C, traditional mineral ascorbates, or natural C supplements may result in flatulence and discomfort with limited absorption. However, modern science has discovered a new process that gives Vitamin C a different "molecular personality," solving the problem of sending vital nutrients like Vitamin C *"down the drain."*

Ester C is a non-acidic, naturally (not chemically) processed, patented super-nutrient. An ordinary ascorbate is ascorbic acid reacted with a mineral. Ester C Polyascorbate is a mega-molecular complex mixture made up of ascorbic acid molecules fully reacted with a vital mineral. Ester C Polyascorbate has the same neutral pH as distilled water and is so gentle that *superior absorption* is possible! I recommend at least 3,000 mg daily, more if you have been ill.

During the exclusive natural process, some of the Vitamin C in Ester C undergoes structural changes into various forms called metabolites. Some researchers believe these metabolites are the key to enhancing blood and tissue levels of Vitamin C. Since neither the food we eat, nor the Vitamin C supplements we take, contain more than trace levels of these metabolites, it is clear why Ester C is the superior source of bioavailable Vitamin C. Ester C Polyascorbate with naturally occurring metabolites is *the key to the power of Vitamin C.*

A, D, E—The Fat Soluble Vitamins

Vitamin A is a fat-soluble vitamin; i.e., the presence of fat is necessary in the diet for Vitamin A to be properly absorbed by the intestines. Chronic alcohol ingestion results in the liver's decreased ability to store vitamin A in the liver, actually leading to a deficiency.

Vitamin D, the sunshine vitamin, is also a member of the fat-soluble vitamin family. Exposure of the skin to the sunshine produces Vitamin D, which is then absorbed into the body. The primary place of storage is in the liver. Vitamin D is necessary for the body to properly utilize calcium and phosphorus which are important for strong bones and teeth.

Vitamin E is also a fat-soluble vitamin. Fat metabolism disturbances might occur after many years of alcohol ingestion that limit the absorption of Vitamin E. Vitamin E's most important function is as an antioxidant, and this is especially important to the alcoholic. Vitamin E also plays a role in the protection of vitamin A, as well as fats and oils.

The Minerals

While minerals comprise only four to five percent of the body's total weight, these "elements" are very powerful substances. Vitamins *cannot* function without the assistance of the minerals. Minerals work together as a group rather than individually. They work in conjunction with hormones, enzymes, proteins, amino acids, carbohydrates, fats, and vitamins. The body requires minerals for the proper overall mental and physical functioning and to build and maintain the body structure.

Calcium is the most abundant mineral found in the body. While 99% of the calcium is found in bones and teeth, the other 1% is in the soft tissues and blood. This 1% has a great effect on the nerves. A double-blind study with anxiety-prone patients and normal patients showed strong similarities between the symptoms of an anxiety attack and the mental effects of calcium deficiency, thus further evidence of the importance of calcium in mental health.

Magnesium is the stress mineral. Over the past several years the focus has been on calcium for the prevention and treatment of osteoporosis, to lower high blood pressure, and to keep muscles in the body operating properly. Few people, if any, know that magnesium is needed for the same reason plus many more. In the process of trying to get sufficient amounts of calcium, most people pay little attention to their intake of magnesium.

Like calcium, magnesium also helps ensure you have strong bones and teeth, lowers high blood pressure, and maintains muscle health. *While calcium is needed for muscle contraction, magnesium is required for muscle relaxation.* Some recent research shows magnesium is needed in a balance of 2 parts magnesium to 1 part calcium.

According to Sherry Rogers, M.D., conditions that may be associated with magnesium deficiency include: gastrointestinal disorders such as malabsorption syndromes due to bowel resection, prolonged diarrhea, alcoholic cirrhosis, and pancreatitis. Other conditions associated with magnesium deficiency include anxiety and panic attacks, osteoarthritis, depression, hyperactivity, eclampsia, premenstrual syndrome, hyperthyroidism, insomnia, cardiovascular disease, excessive perspiration, and body odor. Diuretic therapy, caffeine or soda ingestion, excessive lactation, renal disease, and endocrine disorders also have magnesium deficiency reports.

Many people have spastic conditions clearly caused by a deficiency of magnesium. These conditions include asthma, migraine, colitis, angina, chronic back pain, muscle spasms, arrhythmias, vasculitis, hypertension, eye twitches, cystitis, tremors, sleep disorders, seizures, Raynaud's disease, infertility, and nystagmus. But vertigo (dizziness), psychosis, confusion, eclampsia, diabetes, phlebitis, exhaustion, T.I.A.'s (transient spasms of arteries in head), refractoriness to potassium therapy, and insulin can also be due to magnesium deficiency.

All patients with anxiety and panic attacks at the Pain & Stress Center are put on magnesium. Usually Mag Link or Mag Chlor 85 Liquid is used, and improvement is felt within 48 hours. Mag Link and Mag Chlor 85 are both, magnesium chloride. Magnesium chloride is efficiently absorbed in the alkaline area of the small intestine. Taking magnesium supplements does not cause a problem with adverse reaction unless you have kidney disease. The kidneys can compensate for an excess uptake by increasing urinary excretion of magnesium.

I have found that my body requires six Mag Link per day, spaced throughout the day. The most common side effect from magnesium supplementation is loose stools or diarrhea. This is welcome relief for anyone who has suffered from chronic constipation. You must be patient and find your body's optimal dose. In addition, Mag Chlor 85 Liquid, 10 to 25 drops, twice to three times daily in juice or water provides additional magnesium. Mag Chlor is the most concentrated liquid magnesium available. Take the magnesium up to bowel tolerance, or loose stools. If loose stools occur, decrease your dose by one Mag Link or 5 drops of Mag Chlor.

Most people short change themselves in magnesium, along with other critically needed nutrients. Although the D.V. (Daily Value) for magnesium is 400 mg, the typical American diet supplies between 200-300 mg daily.

Many patients ask what test they could run to find out just how deficient they are. Blood tests like C.B.C. (complete blood count) or R.B.C. (red blood cell) magnesium and the plasma magnesium are practically useless. In most people the test comes back normal, yet the person exhibits magnesium deficiency signs and symptoms. These tests miss about 80 percent of the people deficient in magnesium.

Dr. Jon Pangborn suggests if specific amino acids are low in a amino acid analysis, you can be pretty sure you have a magnesium deficiency. Magnesium levels can also be determined with collection of a 24-hour urine. Then load challenges of magnesium are given and another 24-hour urine is collected for analysis of magnesium uptake and excretion. So urine, not blood, will be the true test of how much magnesium the body needs.

One of the most common symptoms of magnesium deficient patients is chronic back and neck pain. Since I began using it for an old auto accident whiplash, I have felt 100 percent improvement. For patients in a great deal of pain, we use I.V. magnesium to bring relief from painful muscle spasms. Magnesium deficiency is one of the causes of protracted muscle spasms, stiff and sore muscles upon awakening, and anxiety.

Magnesium deficiency causes the body to release more histamine. Histamine is released whenever you react to an allergen which triggers an allergic reaction—whether environmental, chemical, or food related. A reaction to a food can trigger symptoms that mimic an anxiety attack.

Life is said to begin at 40, but I'm afraid the same cannot be said of bone mass. At the age of 35, after reaching its peak, bone mass starts to decline due to an imbalance of the modeling process, and bones start to lose both their mineral and their gelatinous matrix. Women in menopause, or change of life, begin a bone crisis. At this time a rapid decrease in bone mass occurs. Thus, we see women sustaining more fractures than those taking a regular supplement program that includes enough magnesium.

In summary, remember several major points. As with many minerals, the average diet is deficient in magnesium. The diet only provides 40 percent of the D.V. Dr. Mildred Seelig, a nationally recognized magnesium specialist, estimates deficiencies in over 80 percent of the population. Given all of the available research done, you should certainly reevaluate your current health status and add needed magnesium. If you have kidney disease, consult your doctor.

Potassium is vital for the proper functioning of nerves, heart, and muscles; in addition, it works with sodium to maintain the body's water/salt balance. Potassium deficiency symptoms include muscular fatigue, lack of appetite, and mental apathy. Hypoglycemia (low blood sugar) causes a loss of potassium; hypoglycemia seems to be present in many alcoholics.

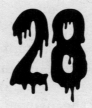

28

I blew the silent whistle again.

And turned to the window. *Buster, where are you?*

The gnomes must have been asking the same question. Because they froze in place, too. The excited chattering, giggling, and chanting stopped.

The only sound I could hear was my own shallow breathing.

I stared up at the window. A rectangle of blackness. No sign of Buster.

"Hey!" Moose's cry made me turn around.

"Look at them!" Moose's voice echoed through the silence.

"Look — they all froze!" Mindy declared. She placed both hands on the orange hat of a gnome — and pushed the gnome over.

It clattered to the floor. And didn't move. A hunk of plaster.

"I don't get it!" Moose scratched his crew cut.

Still gripping the dog whistle tightly, I moved around the room, examining the frozen gnomes, pushing them over. Enjoying the silence.

"Back in their trance state," Mindy murmured.

"But *how*?" Moose demanded. "Buster never showed up. If they weren't terrified of the dog, why did they all freeze up again?"

I suddenly knew the answer. I raised the whistle and blew it again. "It was the whistle," I explained. "It wasn't Buster. I had it wrong. They were afraid of the whistle. Not the dog."

"Let's get out of here," Mindy said softly. "I never want to see another lawn gnome as long as I live."

"Wait till I tell my parents about this!" Moose declared.

"Whoa!" I cried, grabbing his shoulder. "We can't tell *anyone* about this. No way!"

"Why not?" he demanded.

"Because no one will believe it," I replied.

Moose stared at me for a long moment. "You're right," he agreed finally. "You're definitely right."

Mindy moved to the wall and stared up at the window. "How do we get out of here?"

"I know how," I told her. I picked up Hap and Chip and stood them beneath the window. Then I climbed onto their shoulders, lifted my hands to the window, and pulled myself up. "Thanks for the boost, guys!" I called down.

(premenstrual syndrome).

Contemporary researchers and physicians are confirming the conclusions contained in medical texts more than 1,500 years old that praise the anti-inflammatory, anti-arthritic, and anti-pain applications of the gummy extract of a tree commonly found in India.

Researchers and clinicians are showing that Boswellia effectively shrinks inflamed tissue, the underlying cause of pain in many conditions. Boswellia also improves the blood supply to the affected area, and promotes, repair of local blood vessels damaged from proliferating inflammation.

In the United States, physicians are giving Boswellia high marks for effectiveness. They have reported success among hundreds of patients suffering from a variety of advanced muscular and skeletal conditions for which other treatments failed to help.

Boswellia helps patients with arthritis, fibromyalgia, muscle pain of all types, degenerative joint disease following traumatic injuries, muscle wasting and loss of function, knee, foot, and ankle disease; and low-back pain with radiation down the leg.

Antonio Ruiz, M.D., Medical Director of the Pain and Stress Center, states that many patients with a variety of stress-induced soft-tissue pain conditions, such as fibrositis and occupational cumulative trauma disorders, are reporting substantial relief with Boswellia. These are normally elusive problems to treat. Patients are very pleased with the results and report they experience no side effects or discomfort.

Many of my female patients find Boswellia also effective for symptoms associated with perimenopause and P.M.S. The benefits are enhanced with the addition of another well-known Indian herb, ashwagandha. Ashwagandha produces a calming effect in the body, and boosts immunity and stamina. Women who hurt all over, get headaches, do not sleep well, and suffer from fatigue are getting real help. Usual dosage of Boswellia Plus is 300 mg, twice to four times daily, divided.

Pain Control Cream is an advanced pain relief cream that provides fast, lasting relief for overworked or knotted muscles, stress-tension aches and pains, or overused joints. Many anxiety sufferers have muscle tension pain. Pain Control Cream contains bromelain, emu oil, boswellia, glucosamine sulfate, MSM, and pregnenolone. When you apply Pain Control Cream to the skin, it penetrates the skin quickly for prompt relief.

Ginger. Imagine a drug in the arsenal of modern medicine that can simultaneously relieve pain, moderate blood stickiness or aggregation, help digestion, kill parasites, diminish cramps, and reduce the symptoms of a cold. What drug, either in trial or approved by the FDA, can rival indomethacin as an anti-inflammatory, aspirin as an antipyretic, codeine as an antitussive, metoclopromide as an antiemetic, and cimetidine as an antiulcer agent? Imagine such a drug without side effects. There is no such drug, but there is a common root that fits this description. Over the past 30 years, scientific research has not only confirmed the validity of medical applications, but it has begun to uncover how ginger works.

For earaches, headaches, stomach aches, joint aches—whatever aches both internally and externally—ginger has been historically the herb of choice. Ginger is the quintessential digestive herb, whether the need is to restore balance (heal an ulcer, chase a parasite, relieve nausea) or realize full digestive potential (encourage friendly flora growth, enhance bioavailability, protect liver function). In one animal study, ginger was found to confer a 97.5 percent protection factor against stress-induced ulcers. In one group of studies it was found that four major groups of parasites, including the larvae that reside in sushi, were either inhibited or destroyed by ginger. No matter the source of nausea—from ocean travel to pregnancy—studies demonstrate a significant antiemetic activity for ginger.

Recent studies show ginger's potent activity against two causes of nausea: morning sickness and anesthesia. The first study appeared in the *European Journal of Obstetrics and Gynecology and Reproductive Biology* (1990) and dealt with the most severe form of morning sickness. Daily doses of ginger powder given over a four-day period were effective against this condition. Modern allopathic medicine offers no safe remedies for morning sickness because medicating the mother medicates the fetus as well. FDA-approved nausea-reducing drugs are strong sedatives with serious side effects.

On the proactive side, ginger's most important contributions come from its enzyme activity and biopotentiation effects. It is not a coincidence that ginger has been included in a majority of traditional oriental formulations. Recent research has shown it has the ability to increase drug bio-availability by as much as 100 percent.

Four hundred constituents have been isolated from ginger, some of which have been linked to its digestive properties. Ginger contains at least six antiulcer constituents, multiple enzymes, pungent compounds, and a complex interplay of elements that affect how the body uses serotonin in the digestive tract.

One of the lesser-known, yet potentially most important, applications of ginger is as a heart tonic. A review of the research suggests that it could be equal in value to other, better-known cardiotonic herbs such as garlic and hawthorn. Studies also suggest that, used in conjunction with these herbs, ginger might augment their efficacy.

The mechanism for this action is most likely attributable to modulation of prostaglandins. In addition to this phenomenal aspirin-like effect, ginger offers extraordinary antioxidant properties, a cardiotonic effect similar to digitalis, and a potential to lower serum cholesterol.

The Hormones

DHEA (Dehydroepiandrosterone), a steroid hormone produced by the adrenal glands, is considered a key bio-marker in determining biological age. DHEA blood levels peak in our mid-twenties, but decline precipitously as the body ages. By the time we reach our sixties, DHEA levels are barely detectable. Levels measure lower in individuals with medical disease conditions compared to "healthy" individuals the same age. I start my patients on 25 mg of DHEA at age 40 and 50 mg at age 50.

The body produces DHEA in larger amounts than any other adrenal steroid hormone. DHEA functions as a precursor to the sex hormones and as a "buffer" hormone. Stress and anxiety burn available DHEA faster than normal.

Julian M. Whitaker, M.D., editor of *Health and Healing*, states "Supplemental DHEA has therapeutic potential for many medical conditions, including:

- Cardiovascular disease
- Diabetes
- Hypercholesterolemia
- Obesity
- Cancer
- Alzheimer's disease
- Memory deficits
- Parkinson's disease
- Autoimmune diseases and immune disorders including AIDS, Multiple Sclerosis, Chronic Fatigue, and Osteoporosis.

Supplemental DHEA is currently being used clinically for these conditions, as well as for physical and psychological well-being and life extension. In addition, DHEA has been shown to:

- Enhance resistance to infection, through increased antibody effects.
- Decrease the stickiness of platelets (small particles in the

blood that often clump together and cause heart attacks and strokes).

- Lower blood pressure in animals.
- Increase the level of estrogen in women and testosterone in men to levels found in younger men and women.

Pregnenolone is a super hormone neurosteroid synthesized from cholesterol, the primary raw material in the body. Converted into a multitude of steroids and neurosteroids, Pregnenolone is the parent steroid in humans from which all other steroids derive. Pregnenolone has the ability to keep the brain functioning at peak capacity and is believed by scientists to be the most potent memory enhancer of all time.

Pregnenolone, produced in the brain and adrenal cortex, plays an important role in the many aspects of cellular controls. William Regelson, M.D., a professor of medicine at the Medical College of Virginia and author of the best-seller *The Superhormone Promise*, describes extensive research dating back to the 1940s about the benefits of pregnenolone. Dr. Regelson believes pregnenolone not only potently enhances memory, but also improves concentration, fights mental fatigue, relieves arthritis pain, and aids with depression.

The first studies on pregnenolone were done by Hans Selye, a neuroendocrinologist and father of the stress response and its effects on the body. Dr. Selye's research established that with the decline in age, continued stress, and/or disease, pregnenolone levels continue to drop. This drop leads to a decreased capacity to cope with daily stress and increased environmental toxins. By the time a person reaches the age of seventy-five, he makes sixty percent less pregnenolone than someone in his thirties.

Dr. Regelson noted that as pregnenolone level drops, so does production of the other hormones in the steroid pathway. "Since pregnenolone is the parent hormone from which other hormones are made, this makes perfect sense." Dr. Regelson believes pregnenolone and DHEA create an excellent combination to prevent age-related declines of super hormones, since they work in harmony.

Pregnenolone enhances the overworked adrenals and has the capability to assist in repair of the myelin sheath membrane that protects the brain and nervous system. Pregnenolone's influence on brain function is extensive and vitally important. In a recent study completed by The National Institute of Mental Health (NIMH), results showed people with clinical depression have abnormally low levels of pregnenolone in their cerebral spinal fluid. The cause for depression seems to lie in the nerve cells in the brain that must withstand a constant bombardment of stressful stimuli.

GABA, a major inhibitor neurotransmitter, cools and protects the brain and nerve cells from burning out from prolonged stress. Research by NIH demonstrates that pregnenolone moderates the effect of GABA and helps restore the neurotransmitter balance in the brain. Eugene Roberts, Ph.D., a leading researcher in neurochemistry at Washington University in St. Louis and the scientist who discovered the amazing amino acid GABA, states pregnenolone has excitatory effects on membranes such as neurotransmitters.

Dr. Roberts' research disclosed that one milligram of pregnenolone given before bedtime has been reported to increase the amount of slow-wave sleep relative to total sleep. Interestingly, his research also disclosed the amygdala as the most sensitive brain region for memory enhancement by pregnenolone or other substances such as DHEA, glutamine, and phosphatidylserine. Although much of the focus regarding pregnenolone has been on memory and brain function, it has the potential for a major pain reliever.

In *The Superhormone Promise,* Dr. Regelson reports that pregnenolone was used in the 1940s with a great deal of success as a treatment for rheumatoid arthritis, an autoimmune disease. Even though pregnenolone had great potential as a major pain reducer, the research stopped in the 1940s. The major reason that research was not continued is that pregnenolone is a natural substance and could not be patented. The drug companies were not interested in a research investment because they could not see the big profits they require.

Dr. Roberts reports some of the original pregnenolone studies regarding arthritis continued for two years, and during that time no adverse side effects or counter indications were noted. Pregnenolone has a great potential for the millions who suffer from chronic pain without the harmful side effects of drugs.

Pregnenolone has been safe and effective at doses of 25 to 200 mg. If you are taking prescribed steroid hormones, consult your physician before making the change. When pregnenolone and DHEA are taken together they promote only minimal anabolic and estrogenic activity. Research studies recently published demonstrate pregnenolone helps protect against the potential consequences of elevated cortisol, which includes hot flashes, skin atrophy, osteoporosis, and adult-onset diabetes.

Pregnenolone, DHEA, and melatonin are all considered "biomarkers" of the aging process that usually begins to show around the ages of 35 to 40. All three hormones peak in your twenties, and then begin a rapid decline with each passing year. The physical and mental effects of aging depend on your life-style and, most importantly, stress and how you cope with it. The aging process itself can be slowed; studies point to a strong immune system with its use of antioxidants, the brain with enhanced neurotransmitters, and super hormones for the adrenals.

Melatonin is a potent immune regulator, and is contained in the pineal gland, situated in the anterior portion, at the base of the brain. This gland's main hormone is melatonin. Melatonin has been the subject of intense research in Europe and the U.S.A. The main focus that attracted so much attention is that melatonin metabolizes in the brain as tryptophan and elevates the serotonin level.

Melatonin regulates our biological clock and of the body's circadian rhythm that makes us sleep at night and wake up in the morning. Some researchers consider melatonin a primary regulator of the body's immune system protecting us from all forms of stress. Melatonin's sedative qualities have been shown to decrease anxiety, panic disorders, and some migraine headaches.

Serafina Corsello, an orthomolecular physician, uses melatonin to treat her patients. Dr. Corsello finds melatonin to be one of the most effective interventions in her practice. Patients have reported excellent results for sleep problems. Melatonin is available in 1, 2, or 3 mg capsules. One capsule, an hour before bed, helps alleviate insomnia.

Additional Support Products

TL-Vite is a one-a-day multiple vitamin that provides your body all the basic nutrients it needs to help you through the day.

Liquid Serotonin is a 1X homeopathic formulation for acute stress or anxiety. When the serotonin level in the brain is depleted from stress, anxiety, depression, hyperactivity, or A.D.D., communication in the brain, through neurotransmitters, decreases. Serotonin is one of the neurotransmitters in the brain that helps us feel calm and relaxed. Symptoms of anxiety, tension, depression, and hyperactivity respond to an increase of serotonin in the brain. Liquid Serotonin can be used at any time and by all ages. For prolonged effectiveness, use Liquid Serotonin in conjunction with amino acids for prolonged effectiveness. Recommended dosage: ten to fifteen drops, two to four times daily, as needed. For best results, combine Liquid Serotonin with an amino acid formulation such as Anxiety Control or Mood Sync.

Huperzine A. After years of extensive research and clinical testing. Huperzine A is the active alkaloid extracted, then purified from a rare type of club moss that grows in the cool, mountainous regions of China. Huperzine A is not a drug, but a nutraceutical.

In clinical studies patients with varying degrees of memory

impairment demonstrated a marked improvement using Huperzine A. Prolonged stress, anxiety, grief, or depression can cause memory impairment. If acetylcholine is in short supply due to stress and anxiety, or malnourished brain cells, memory storage and retrieval becomes increasingly difficult. Huperzine A is safe and effective. The recommended dosage is one capsule, morning and evening.

MSM (Methyl Sulfonyl Methane) is a combination of the sulfur-containing amino acids, cysteine, methionine, and taurine. Dr. Stanley Jacob at the University of Oregon researched and developed MSM. Dr. Jacob treated over 12,000 patients over several years with 2,000 mg of MSM daily with excellent results. We use MSM at the Pain & Stress Center for patients with chronic pain and fibromyalgia. Our results have been outstanding. MSM alleviates pain associated with inflammatory disorders, arthritis, muscle spasms, stiffness, and soreness. Patients with migraines reported relief after seven days, and no adverse side effects.

I began taking MSM for my own chronic pain. I could not believe how much better I felt in 48 hours—the difference was remarkable. You can include it in your orthomolecular program. Stress and anxiety causes pain. The pain in and of itself, causes depression, fear, and uncertainty because you do not understand why you hurt, and fear the worst. Many safe and helpful products are available today. *No one should suffer or turn to toxic prescription drugs.*

Celadrin, a revolutionary compound, contains esterified fatty acid carbons that reduce inflammation. Studies in the *Journal of Rheumatology,* found Celadrin, when taken orally, dramatically improved joint and muscle mobility. Celadrin enhances and lubricates the membranes in the body that cushion and protect your bones and joints. Celadrin provides temporary relief of arthritis, minor aches and pains associated with back strain, bruises, and sprains *without side effects.* Celadrin is available in soft gels and as a cream. The recommended dosage is 3 soft gels, twice to three times daily as needed. You can apply the Celadrin cream as needed.

Warning Note: Do not use Celadrin if you are taking anticoagulants (blood thinners such as Coumadin)

Essential Fatty Acids (EFAs) play an important role in anxiety and mood disorders. Lipids (fat) comprises 60% of the solid brain tissues, and alterations of these fats in the tissues influences brain function. Epidemiological studies show that countries with the highest consumption of omega 3 fatty acids have a lower rate of depression. Use Arctic Omega or Pure Fish Oil, 3,000 to 4,000 mg daily.

The Healing Mind

The mind and body are one. There is *no such thing as a purely mental or physical disease.* All disease has a mental and physical component. Dr. Candace Pert, formerly at the NIMH, discovered the GABA receptors as well as many other peptide receptors in the brain and body. This research led to the understanding of the chemicals that travel between the mind and body. Dr. Pert, in an interview with Bill Moyers on the *Healing and the Mind* series, stated, "Your mind is in every cell of your body. Emotions are stored in your body. Everything you do is run by your emotions. The mind is more than the brain. It enables the cells to talk to each other. Neurotransmitters and neuropeptides that are made up of amino acids are the biochemical correlates of emotion. Neurotransmitters and neuropeptides are the chemical messengers that mastermind how the systems of the body talk to each other." Dr. Pert believes moods and attitudes that come from the realm of the mind transform themselves into the physical realm through emotions. Moyer's book, *Healing and the Mind,* opens the door to a new understanding in healing.

Recently, scientists have demonstrated evidence that hormones and neurotransmitters can and do influence the activities of the immune system, and that those same products of the immune system can influence the brain. Dr. David Felten, M.D., at the University of

Rochester School of Medicine, established that there is a constant flow of information that goes back and forth between the brain and the immune system. Hormones are continuously being produced and released, and neurotransmitters are continuously talking to target cells throughout the body. Emotions such as grief, loneliness, chronic depression, and fear can not only change, but also diminish the effectiveness of the immune system. Chronic anxiety, fear, or panic, flood the body and brain with an excess of stress hormones which can lead to the gradual death of some of the brain cells. Brain cells must have food in the form of amino acids that create neurotransmitters that slow down the delicate limbic system. Remember, drugs only use *available* neurotransmitters. They do not create new ones. The progression of healing continues when we address the needs of our brain and body. *Your brain contains every drug you will ever need. We can heal from within. The power of the mind is the power of our whole being.*

XII
Closing Comments

Twenty-one years have passed since I wrote the first edition of *The Anxiety Epidemic*. This has been a time of discovery and learning, a time of reinforcement that prescription drugs are not the answer to anxiety, panic, or fear and they never will be! I thank God for the courage to keep fighting and the strength to keep searching for natural alternatives to help those who walk the lonely path as I once did.

As for all those patients whose symptoms I described on previous pages, they are all healed and live in peace. I am especially happy for Sister Karen. She is now Mother Superior in a very large convent. She has not experienced any more of the old problems, but in times of prolonged stress, she keeps her neurotransmitter formulas handy. Sister Karen had a major deficiency of amino acids and magnesium. She was as depleted as I was after my traumatic years.

A therapist's life is always busy. Although I enjoy my work, it is very demanding. I keep myself on an amino acid and nutrient regime, take time for meditation, and never, ever forget my magnesium. If I had known the problems a magnesium deficiency can cause, I could have avoided so much suffering.

Over the past years, I have seen a multitude of patients from all walks of life, with anxiety, panic, fear, and phobias. They all feel their symptoms are unique, and no one else could suffer as much as they have. Little do they know. Most of them had given in to what they thought would be freedom from anxiety—prescription drugs. What they found out was that they were living in a chemical straightjacket of prescribed addiction.

The pharmaceutical industry, the world's most profitable business, promises new life, and no fear and anxiety, if you will just take their pills. Their power and influence is awesome. They thrive on human illness and weakness, not health and well being.

Antidepressants and tranquilizers do not provide the answer to stress-induced pain, anxiety, depression, grief, or fear. One of the biggest challenges you will face is constantly being offered prescription drugs by well-meaning physicians who think they are helping you. When I think about what would have happened to me and how my life would have turned out if I had not had the courage to say no to the prescription drugs, I know someone was watching over me.

With the Lord's help, I have been able to continue my research and product development to help the thousands who have reached out for help. All the drugs in the world will not put a face on fear, or resolve anxiety. Your life becomes an endless search for answers. The right amino acids and nutrient program, and finding a therapist with *empathic* understanding, will give you your key to a safe, long-term recovery.

As my own search began for answers to my pain and suffering, it ended with a new direction in my life. I have fulfilled my impossible dream because I am living it. I won't deny that there have been times when the past tried to sneak in and pull me back. It has, many times, especially during the holidays. I don't have anxiety or panic attacks anymore, only twinges of grief. I do find myself wondering what my life would have been like if I had not been burned at fourteen months and lost my father at age six. I had a very abusive stepfather who constantly rejected me, and mistreated my mother. I have worked very hard to deal with the emotional pain and let it go, and I have, for the most part. But I still feel the grief, especially when I wonder what I might have felt when calling someone Dad, or handing my first business card to my mother. Then I return to the present, hearing the words, "Peace be with you; now go and do what you have chosen."

Dominus vobiscum.

"Undefeated only because we have gone on trying."

T.S. Eliot

Inadequate Nutrition

BODY SYSTEM	SIGNS & SYMPTOMS	NUTRIENT DEFICIENCY
Mental Central Nervous System (CNS)	Apathy, irritability, psychomotor changes	Protein amino acids
	Aggressive behavior, anger, argumentative, loss of focus, depression, mood swings, OCD	Serotonin (5-HTP), Mood Sync, HTP10, SBNC, L–T
	Dementia, senile changes, psychotic behavior	B12, folic acid, NeuroLinks, Mood Sync, L–T, B6
	Tremors, tics, seizures	B6, magnesium, taurine, GABA
Musculoskeletal	Fibromyalgia, muscle spasms, trigger points, muscle contraction (tension) headaches, stiffness, tender points throughout the body, migraines, TMJ For more information on Fibromyalgia, read my book, *Malic Acid and Magnesium for Fibromyalgia and Chronic Pain Syndrome*	Magnesium chloride such as Mag Link, Mag Chlor 85, Malic Acid Plus, DLPA, Boswellia Plus, Pain Control, Celadrin Soft gels and Cream, Ester C, Essential Fatty Acids (EFAs) such as Pure Omega 3 Fish Oil
	Inflammation of muscles and joints, arthritis, osteoporosis, swelling in legs not related to heart	Magnesium chloride such as Mag Link or Mag Chlor 85, glucosamine, chrondroitin, Ester C, DLPA, Boswellia Plus, Pain Control Cream, Celadrin soft gels and cream, (EFAs) such as Pure Omega 3 Fish Oil
Gastrointestinal	Irritable bowel, digestive problems, gas, diarrhea or constipation, ulcers, anorexia	Digestive enzymes, especially pancreatin, bromelain, zinc, glutamine, mag chloride, B vitamins, AC24, Colon Balance

Skin	Acne, psoriasis, dermatitis, herpes, dry, red spots	Vitamin A, C, E, B12, lysine, zinc, MSM, Pantothenic acid, emu oil, EFAs such as Pure Omega 3 Fish Oil
	Pallor, jaundice	B12
	Bruising, bleeding into joints	Ester C, E
	White spots on face, white and blackheads along border of nose and cheeks	Essential fatty acids, B6
	Sore, cracked and chapped lips; inflammation of the mucus membranes	Riboflavin
	Canker sores	B Complex, topical lysine with zinc,
	Oily skin, hair	lysine, magnesium, Vitamins A & D
	Itching skin, numbness and tingling	B Complex, essential fatty acids (EFAs)
	Hypertrophy or overgrowth of gum, inflammation of gums, purple tongue	Iron, Vitamins C, E Vitamin C, A,
	Red, painful, sore tongue	Niacin, Riboflavin
	Raw, scarlet tongue	B6, Folic Acid
Eyes	Extreme sensitivity to light, poor twilight vision, loss of shine, bright and moist appearance, loss of light reflex, decreased tears, softening of the cornea	Niacin Vitamin A
Nails	Ridging, brittle, easily broken, flattened, dry, thin, lusterless	B Complex, Folic acid, Vitamin C, calcium, zinc, iron, protein,
Cardiovascular (Heart)	Rapid heartbeat, irregular beats, arrhythmias, mitral valve prolapse, high blood pressure, EKG changes, congestive heart failure	Magnesium chloride, folic acid, CoQ10, Taurine, garlic, Carnitine, Vitamin E, C, Scavengers
	High cholesterol, triglycerides	Carnitine, chromium picolinate, red yeast rice, pomegranate, fiber, decrease sugar (carbs) in diet

Kidney	Kidney stones	Magnesium chloride, Vitamins A, E, C, B6, B2
	Kidney disease	Carnitine, BCAA
Other	Shingles (Herpes Zoster), especially in acute stages	Large doses of B12 (Best if IM (intramuscular), + Magnesium chloride (Mag Link), Vitamin C, Lysine, D-Lenolate (Olive Leaf Extract), Vitamins A, E, B6, MSM capsules, Pain Control Cream, emu oil, Celadrin soft gels and cream, EFAs
	Rhinitis, inflamed nasal mucosa	Ester C, NAC, EFAs (3–4 gm fish oil) daily, Vitamin A, MSM capsules
	Hypoglycemia	Chromium pic, biotin, B6, magnesium chloride (Mag Link), B complex, decaf green tea extract, folic acid, carnitine, antioxidants and pomegranate, EFAs, blood sugar balance
	Diabetes	Hypoglycemia supps + vanadium, gymnema sylvestre, niacinamide, lipoic acid, DHEA, fortified flax
	Constipation, hemorrhoids	Magnesium chloride (Mag Link or Mag Chlor 85) fortified flax, Ester C, fiber
Immune	Chronic fatigue, sleep disorder, depression, headaches, anxiety, stiffness, dizziness, joint pain, dry eyes and mouth, night sweats, painful lymph nodes	Brain Link, large amounts of Ester C, flax, CoQ10, decaf green tea extract,

Note: Where Vitamin C is recommended, use Ester C for better tolerance and absorption.

Immune (continued)		mag chloride (Mag Link or Mag Chlor), T-L Vite, DHEA (if over 40), MSM, Mood Sync, Alpha KG
		Magnesium chloride, Sleep Link, Ashwagandha (Mellow Mind), 5-HTP, melatonin, Liquid Serotonin
		EFAs (3–4 gm pure fish oil), Ester C, Beta Glucan, beta carotene NAC (NA Cysteine), MSM, Heel sinus, Sinus & Allergy spray. Euphorium spray. XClear spray. Investigate food allergies.
Thyroid	Low thyroid or symptoms of low thyroid. Most Americans (95%) are very low in iodine.	Supplement with Lugol's solution or Indoral® daily.
Over 40		Consider DHEA and pregnenolone, antioxidants such as decaf green tea extract, Vitamins C, E, pomegranate

Food Reactions

Reactions to foods can cause a wide variety of symptoms ranging from anxiety, migraines to eczema. According to the *Annuals of Allergy* (Vol. 62, 1988, p. 261) researchers estimate sixty percent of Americans suffer from some reaction to a food that can cause or complicate a health problem. Unfortunately, many health care practitioners do not consider foods as a major contributing factor.

Two types of reactions occur to foods—immediate (Type 1–IgE) and delayed (Types II and II–IgG4). Immediate reactions occur within three hours after eating. High IgE antibody blood levels produce immediate allergic reactions exhibiting as *classic* and obvious allergy reactions familiar to many people, such as rash after eating or difficulty breathing. But low levels can go unnoticed, but can over time, cause symptoms.

Delayed reactions or hidden food allergies are much more difficult to notice because they often occur hours or days after

Food Allergy Symptoms

Head and Neck: Recurrent ear infections, watery/itchy eyes, constant runny or stuffy nose, chronic sinus problems, headaches, migraines, sore throat, sneezing, dark circles under eyes.

Nervous System: Mood swings, anxiety, depression, food cravings, poor concentration, fatigue, hyperactivity, nervousness, mental confusion.

Chest: Asthma, irregular heartbeat, rapid pulse increasing greater than 15 points after eating, difficulty breathing.

Digestion: Upset stomach, nausea, diarrhea, constipation, gas, bloating, ulcers, cramps, bad breath, and malabsorption/maldigestion.

Other Symptoms: Water retention, weight gain, hives, rashes, sweating, body aches, stiffness, back, neck, shoulder pains, swelling.

consuming an offending food. Sometimes you may eat a food for several days in a row, then develop a reaction to it. You may not link the reaction to the food and the symptoms—hidden food allergies. High IgG4 antibody blood levels to specific foods are thought to cause these delayed reactions. Often, the offending foods are the foods you love and crave the most. Common offending foods are milk (dairy), corn, wheat, egg, or citrus, but delayed reactions are not limited to these.

What is the answer? Find the offending foods, then eliminate or rotate these foods in your diet. Read labels. Eat the offendng foods *only* every four to five days. For example, when wheat is problematic. Eat wheat on Sunday, then do not eat *wheat in any form* until Thursday or Friday. This allows the body time to elimi-nate the offending foods that cause histamine and antigen release. Over time, your wheat sensitivity can become better.

Conditions Successfully Treated Using Amino Acid Analysis

- Chronic fatigue
- Candida
- Food and chemical sensitivities
- Immune system disorders
- Anxiety
- Depression
- Learning disorders
- A.D.D./hyperactivity
- Behavioral disorders
- Eating disorders
- Cancer
- Hypoglycemia
- Diabetes
- Cardiovascular disease
- Seizures
- Headaches
- Arthritis
- Chronic pain
- Vitamin and mineral deficiencies
- Digestive disorders

For detailed information about amino acid or food allergy testing, call the Pain & Stress Management Clinic at (800) 669-2256 or go to http://www.painstresscenter.com

Amino Acid Testing

Amino acids make up proteins found in every cell of the body and play a major role in almost every chemical process affecting physical and mental functions. Amino acids have more diverse functions than any other nutrients—contributing to the formation of proteins, muscles, neurotransmitters, enzymes, antibodies, and cellular energy production. Amino acid imbalances affect many metabolic processes and can manifest as a variety of clinical symptoms and metabolic disorders.

By utilizing the natural substances in optimal quantities to reestablish a normal balance, you can help correct the cause of some disease processes in a nontoxic way. Amino acid analysis is an analytical technique on the leading edge of nutritional biochemical medicine. It gives a new approach toward illness, and can assist patients who have not responded to treatment as expected, or who present complex cases with diverse symptoms. Amino acid analysis is a tool to determinate amino acid imbalances, evaluation of functional vitamin and mineral deficiencies, and diagnosis of metabolic disorders. For example, fatigue, headache, anxiety, and shakiness between meals can be attributed to deficiencies of specific amino acids. Amino acid analysis measures the levels of amino acids in the body that affect many important processes.

Hypoglycemia, Anxiety, and Panic

Classic hypoglycemia or low blood sugar does not commonly occur. Reactive or functional hypoglycemia occurs more frequently, especially if you have anxiety and panic. Whenever you eat sugar in any form, especially carbohydrates, starches, or sugar, you feel like you get a lift. Your energy increases as your blood sugar rises. The increased blood sugar goes to all parts of your body and brain, including your heart. But this rise is only temporary as your pancreas releases insulin in response to the increased blood glucose (sugar). Insulin helps metabolize or burn the glucose to normalize the blood sugar level.

Ingestion of sweets and other refined carbohydrates stimulates the pancreas to release insulin. If too much insulin is released, hypoglycemia results. A drop in blood glucose to abnormally levels causes symptoms of hypoglycemia including anxiety, panic, and fear. Other symptoms include mood swings, fatigue, depression, headaches, nervousness, irritability, sweating, weakness, sleep disturbances, and shakiness. When you consume a large amount of highly sugared foods, your body begins a yo-yo pattern.

Sugar contributes to many behavior problems including hyperactivity, anxiety, mood swings, depression, and aggression. Many

Blood Sugar Cycle

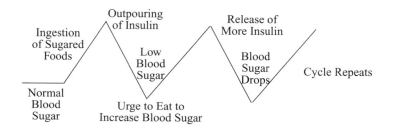

factors should be explored if you have a problem with sugar, you could have an addiction. Look at the power of sugar. Most people say they can give it up at any time if they want to, but they cannot. As you begin to feel more anxious, you reach for something sweet such as a soft drink. The amount of sugar and caffeine in soft drinks intensifies anxiety symptoms. Instead, use the amino acid, Glycine, when you crave sugar. Remember, sugar contributes to increased anxiety and panic, so limit your intake.

Phobia Dictionary

Following is a non-inclusive list of phobias and the fears they represent.

ACHLUOPHOBIA - darkness
ACROPHOBIA - heights
AEROPHOBIA - high objects, heights or flying
AGORAPHOBIA - open places
AGYROPHOBIA - crossing streets
AICHMOPHOBIA - knives
AILUROPHOBIA - cats
ALGIOPHOBIA - pain
AMATHOPHOBIA - dust
ANTHROPOPHOBIA - people
ANTLOPHOBIA - floods
ASTRAPHOBIA - lightning
BATHOPHOBIA - depth
BATOPHOBIA - high buildings
BELONEPHOBIA - needles
CANCERPHOBIA - cancer
CARDIOPHOBIA - heart disease
CIBOPHOBIA - food
CLAUSTROPHOBIA - confinement
CLIMACOPHOBIA - stairs
CYNOPHOBIA - dogs
DECIDOPHOBIA - making decisions
DENTOPHOBIA - dentists
DERMATOSIOPHOBIA - skin disease
DIABETOPHOBIA - Diabetes
DOMATOPHOBIA - being confined in a house
ELECTROPHOBIA - electricity
EMETOPHOBIA - vomiting
ENTOMOPHOBIA - insects
EPISTEMOPHOBIA - learning
EREMOPHOBIA - being alone
GALEOPHOBIA - cats
GEPHYROPHOBIA - crossing bridges
GERONTOPHOBIA - old age
HEMOPHOBIA - blood
HODOPHOBIA - road travel
HORMEPHOBIA - shock
HYDROPHOBIA - water

HYPENGYOPHOBIA - responsibility
IATROPHOBIA - going to doctors
KAINOPHOBIA - change
KAKORRHAPHIOPHOBIA - failure
LALOPHOBIA - speaking in public
LYSSOPHOBIA - insanity
MENINGITOPHOBIA - meningitis
MYSOPHOBIA - germs or contamination and dirt
NECROPHOBIA - dead bodies
NUCLEOMITIPHOBIA - nuclear bombs
NYCTOPHOBIA - night
OCHLOPHOBIA - crowds
OMBROPHOBIA - rain
OPHIDIOPHOBIA, OPHIOPHOBIA - snakes
PANTOPHOBIA - fears
PATHOPHOBIA - disease
PELADOPHOBIA - baldness
PHAGOPHOBIA - eating
PHARMACOPHOBIA - drugs
PHOBOPHOBIA - one's own fears
PNIGEROPHOBIA - smothering
PNIGOPHOBIA - choking
POINEPHOBIA - punishment
PSYCHROPHOBIA - cold
PYROPHOBIA - fire
SCIOPHOBIA - shadows
SCOPOPHOBIA - shyness
SELACHOPHOBIA - sharks
SELAPHOBIA - light flashes
THALASSOPHOBIA - the sea
THANATOPHOBIA - death
THEOPHOBIA - God
TOPOPHOBIA - performing (stage fright)
TREMOPHOBIA - trembling
TROPOPHOBIA - moving or making a change
VACCINOPHOBIA - vaccination
XENOPHOBIA - strangers

You Hold

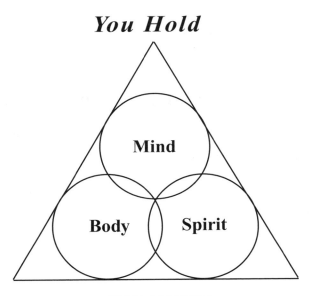

THE KEY!

Your mind, body and spirit are one . . .
You cannot nourish them with toxic prescription drugs.
You must hold firmly in your mind what prescription drugs are,
  and everything they are not . . .
Prescription drugs repress your emotions, nothing gets in to hurt
  or frighten you, but nothing gets out to be resolved.
Drugs can cause emotional sterility.
Your life is influenced by the sufferings that surround you and at
  times envelope you.
Everyday, you see other victims of toxic drug influences.
They are lost in a sea of red, green, and blue pills.
Drugs encourage a passive existence.
Your mind, body and spirit need the nourishment of neurotrans-
  mitters, to heal from the ravages of stress, anxiety, depression,
  and grief.
Feed them with love, understanding, and the natural medicine in
  your brain God gave every one of us.
Let your healing begin!

Product Information

The *purity* of amino acids plays an important part in your success rate. You generally get what you pay for, and this holds true with supplements and amino acids. Be selective. Your body responds to what you absorb. This absorption is enhanced when you *use only pharmaceutical grade products,* and not off brand mixes or blends. Supplements are made of four grades of supplemental amino acids and vitamins and include:

1) Food lot
2) Cosmetic
3) Pharmaceutical grade
4) I.V. grade

Pharmaceutical grade generally guarantees purity of product. Capsules are generally cleaner and purer than tablets, and *more bioavailable.* Tablets require fillers and binders. When considering nutritional supplements, look for preservative-free and excipient-free products because they are better. Purity is important, so buy supplements that are free of preservatives, fillers, binders, or excipients of any kind. *Insist on pharmaceutical grade products.* Your body and brain will know the difference.

What does hypoallergenic mean? Simply, non-allergy producing. Products labeled hypoallergenic means that the product has been formulated and the production is done in such a way to ensure minimum instances of allergic reactions. If you have a problem with allergies, use hypoallergenic products.

For product information, call 1-800-669-2256 or visit
http://www.painstresscenter.com

Other Resources

Anxiety/Panic Attacks CD by Billie J. Sahley, Ph.D.

Anxiety CD, by Billie J. Sahley, Ph.D.

Phobias CD by Billie J. Sahley, Ph.D.

Escape CD by Billie J. Sahley, Ph.D.

Break Your Prescribed Addiction by Drs. Billie. Sahley and K. Birkner

Chronic Emotional Fatigue, by Billie J. Sahley, Ph.D.

GABA, The Anxiety Amino Acid by Billie J. Sahley, Ph.D

Heal with Amino Acids by Drs. Billie Sahley and Kathy Birkner

Inside the Brain by Ronald Kotulak

Malic Acid And Magnesium For Fibromyalgia and Chronic Pain Syndrome by Dr. Billie J. Sahley

Post Trauma and Chronic Emotional Fatigue by Billie J. Sahley, Ph.D.

Therapeutic Use of Amino Acids CD by Billie J. Sahley, Ph.D.

5-HTP, The Natural Serotonin Solution by Richard A. Passwater, Ph.D. and James South, M.A.

The Anti-Depressant Fact Book by Peter R. Breggin, M.D.

Depression Cured at Last by Sherry Rogers, M.D.

Detoxify or Die by Sherry Rogers, M.D.

The E.I. Syndrome by Sherry Rogers, M.D.

Food Allergies Made Simple by Phylis Austin, et al.

The Great Anxiety Escape by Max Ricketts

Molecules of Emotion by Candace Pert, Ph.D.

No More Heartburn by Sherry Rogers, M.D.

Overdose (Prescription Drugs and Your Health) by Jay Cohen, M.D.

Pain Free in 6 Weeks by Sherry Rogers, M.D.

Prozac Backlash by Joseph Glenmullen, M.D.

The Second Brain by Michael D. Gershon, M.D.

Tired or Toxic by Sherry Rogers, M.D

Toxic Psychiatry by Peter R. Breggin, M.D.

Your Drug May Be Your Problem by Peter R. Breggin, M.D.

Consulting

Dr. Sahley is not currently accepting new patients, as she is focusing on research and writing. However, her office does offer consultations with a certified nutritional consultant (C.N.C.) that has been trained by Dr. Sahley at affordable prices. The consultant can help you personalize your nutritional program to help with your specific needs tailoring it to you and your particular needs.

You talk directly with the C.N.C. professional that has experience and expertise in orthomolecular therapy and nutritional supplements. Sessions are personalized and confidential in the privacy of your home or office via telephone or at the Pain & Stress Center in San Antonio. You receive answers to your questions one-on-one and help with your special needs and moving your health toward your wellness goals.

Call 1-800-669-2256 to schedule your consultation today!

Bibliography

Aggleton, John P., ed. *The Amygdala*. New York, NY: Wiley-Liss, Inc., 1992.

Ashmead, DeWayne. "Lead Toxicity." *Health Express*. October 1983, pp. 16–17.

Benson, Herbert. *The Mind/Body Effect*. New York: Simon and Schuster, 1979.

Bergmann, Kenneth J. "Prozabide: A New GABA-Mimetic Agent in Clinical Use." *Clinical Neuropharmacology*. Vol. 8, No. 1, 1985. New York: Raven Press, pp. 13–23.

Birdsall, Timothy C. "5-Hydroxytryptophan: A Clinically-Effective Serotonin Precursor." *Alternative Medicine Review*, Vol. 3, No. 4, 1998, pp. 271-280.

Birkner, Katherine M. *Breaking Your Sugar Habit Cookbook*. San Antonio, TX: Pain & Stress Publications, 1995.

Bland, Jeffrey, ed. *Medical Applications of Clinical Nutrition*. New Canaan, CN: Keats Publishing, Inc., 1983.

Blier, P, et al. "Modifications of the Serotonin System by Antidepressant Treatments: Implications fro the Therapeutic Response in Major Depression." *Journal of Clinical Psychopharmacology*, Vol. 7, 1987, pp. 24S–35S.

Braestrup, Claus, and Mogens Nielsen. "Neurotransmitters and CNS Disease." *The Lancet*. November 1982, pp. 1030–1034.

"The Brain" series. Public Broadcasting Service, January, 1985.

Braverman, Eric R., and Carl C. Pfeiffer. *The Healing Nutrients Within*. New Canaan, CN: Keats Publishing, Inc., 1987.

Breggin, Peter. *Brain Disabling Treatments in Psychiatry*. New York: Springer Publishing Co., 1997.

Breggin, Peter R. *Toxic Psychiatry*. New York, NY: St. Martin's Press, 1991.

Breggin, Peter R., and Ginger Ross Breggin. *Talking Back to Prozac*. New York: St. Martin's Press, 1994.

Bresler, David E., with Richard Trubo. *Free Yourself From Pain*. New York: Simon and Schuster, 1979.

Brown, Barbara. *Between Health and Illness*. New York: Bantam Books, 1985.

Brown, C. C. et al. "Effects of L-Tryptophan on Sleep Onset Insomniacs." *Walking and Sleeping*. April 1979, pp. 101–108.

Callahan, Sheila. "Tension Headaches. What's in a Name?" *Aches and Pains*. October 1980, pp. 14–16.

Carper, Jean. *Stop Aging Now!* New York, NY: HarperCollins Publishers, 1995.

Carter, Rita. *Mapping the Mind*. Berkley, CA: University of California Press, 1998.

Challem, Jack Joseph. "Everything You Need to Know About Amino Acids." *Health Quarterly*. Winter 1982, pp. 13, 60–61.

Chweh, A.Y., et al. "Effect of GABA Agonists on Neurotoxicity and Anticonvulsant Activity of Benzodiazepines." *Life Sciences*. Vol. 36, No. 8, 1985, pp. 737–744.

Cohen, Jay S. *Over Dose*. New York: Jeremy P. Tarcher/Putnam, 2001.

Cohen, Jay S. *Magnesium and Hypertension*. Del Mar, CA: Medical Alternatives That Work, 2002.

Cohen, Jay S. *Magnesium and Migraine Headaches*. Del Mar, CA: Medical Alternatives That Work, 2002

Colby-Morley, Elsa. "Neurotransmitters and Nutrition." *Journal of Orthomolecular Psychiatry*. First Quarter 1983, pp. 38–39.

Cooper, Jack R. et al. *The Biochemical Basis of Neuropharmacology*. 5th Ed. New York: Oxford Press, 1986.

Cowen, P.J. and D. J. Nutt. "Abstinence Symptoms After Withdrawal of Tranquilizing Drugs: Is There a Common Neurochemical Mechanism?" *The Lancet*. August 14, 1982, pp. 360–362.

Diamond, Seymour and Joe L. Medina. "Headaches." *Clinical Symposia*. Vol. 33, No. 2. Summit, NJ: CIBA Pharmaceutical Co., 1981.

Dietrich, Schneider-Helmert. "Interval Therapy with L-Tryptophan in Severe Chronic Insomniacs." *International Pharmaco-psychiatry*. Vol. 16, 1981, pp. 162–173.

Doheny, Kathleen. "Panic Attacks: A Debilitating Disorder for Millions." *Health Express*. June 1983, pp. 60–61.

Downs, Robert, and Alice Van Baak. "The Amazing Power of Amino Acids, Part I." *Bestways*. January 1982, pp. 74–75.

Downs, Robert and Alice Van Baak. "The Amazing Power of Amino Acids, Part II." *Bestways*. February 1982, pp. 56–58.

Dunne, Lavon J. *Nutrition Almanac*. 3rd Ed. New York: McGraw-Hill Publishing Co., 1990.

"Emotions in Pain." *Pain Current Concepts on Pain and Analgesia*. Vol. 5, No. 1, pp. 1–2.

Essman, W.B., ed. *Nutrients and Brain Function*. New York, NY: Karger, 1987.

Ferguson, Marilyn. *The Aquarian Conspiracy, Personal and Social Transformation in the 1980's*. Los Angeles, CA: J. P. Tarcher, Inc., 1980.

Fishman, Scott M. and David V. Sheehan. "Anxiety and Panic: Their Cause and Treatment." *Psychology Today*. April 1985, pp. 26–32.

Fox, Arnold and Barry Fox. *DLPA to End Chronic Pain and Depression*. New York, NY: Pocket Books, 1985.

Garrison, Robert Jr. *Lysine, Tryptophan, and Other Amino Acids*. New Canaan, CN: Keats Publishing, Inc., 1982.

Gelb, Harold. *Killing Pain Without a Prescription*. New York: Harper and Row Publishers, 1980.

Gelenberg, Alan J. et al. "Tyrosine For the Treatment of Depression." *American Journal of Psychiatry*. May 1980, pp. 622–623.

Gershon, Michael D. *The Second Brain*. New York: HarperCollins Publishers, 1998.

Gitlin, Michael J. *The Psychotherapist's Guide to Psycho-pharmacology*. New York, NY: The Free Press, 1990.

Glenmullen, Joseph. *Prozac Backlash*. NY: Simon & Schuster, March, 2000.

Grant, Larry A. "Amino Acids in Action." *Let's Live Magazine*. August 1983, pp. 61–64.

Guyton, Arthur C. *Basic Human Neurophysiology.* Third Edition. Phildelphia: W.B. Saunders Company, 1981, pp. 207–217, 223.

Hammond, Edward J., and B. J. Wilder. "Gamma-Vinyl GABA: A New Antiepileptic Drug. *Clinical Neuropharmacology.* Vol. 8, No. 1, 1985, pp. 1–12.

Health Express, "Stress Reaction," June 1983, p. 48.

Hersen, Michael et al. *Progress in Behavior Modification.* Vol. 14. New York: Academic Press, 1983.

Hoffer, Abram, and Morton Walker. *Orthomolecular Nutrition.* New Canaan, CN: Keats Publishing, Inc., 1978.

Hoffer, Abram and Morton Walker. *Putting It All Together: The New Orthomolecular Nutrition.* New Canaan, CN: Keats Publishing, Inc., 1996.

Iverson, Leslie L. "Neurotransmitters." *The Lancet.* October 23, 1982. pp. 914–918.

Kaplan, Harold I, Freedman, Alfred, and Sadock, Benjamin. *Comprehensive Textbook of Psychiatry.* Vol. 3. Baltimore: Williams and Wilkins, 1980.

King, Robert B. "Pain and Tryptophan." *Journal Neurosurgery 53.* July 1980, pp. 44–52.

Klatz, Ronald M., ed. *Advances in Anti-Aging Medicine.* Volume 1, Larchmont, NY: Mary Ann Liebert, Inc., 1996.

Kolata, Gina. "Your Hungry Brain." *American Health.* May/June 1983, pp. 45–50.

Kotulak, Ronald. *Inside the Brain.* Kansas City, MO: Andrews and McMeel, 1996.

LeDoux, Joseph. "Probing Circuits of Normal and Pathological Fear through Studies of Fear Conditioning." Center for Neuroscience of Fear and Anxiety, Center for Neural Science, New York University, 2002.

LeDoux, Joseph. *Synaptic Self, How Our Brains Become Who We Are.* New York: Penguin Putnam, Inc., 2002.

Lee, William H. "Amazing Amino Acids." New Canaan, CN: Pine Grove Pamphlet Division of Keats Publishing, Inc., 1984.

Leonard, B. E. *Fundamentals of Psychopharmacology.* New York, NY: John Wiley & Sons, 1992.

Lesser, Michael. *Nutrition and Vitamin Therapy.* New York: Bantam Books, 1981.

Locke, Steven, and Douglas Colligan. *The Healer Within.* New York, NY: Signet, 1987.

Lowry, Thomas P. *Hyperventilation and Hysteria.* Springfield, Illinois: Banner Stone House, 1967.

Mann, John et al. "D-Phenylalanine in Endogenous Depression." *American Journal of Psychiatry.* December 1980, pp. 1611–1612.

Mazer, Eileen. "Tryptophan—The Three Way Misery Reliever." *Prevention Magazine.* May 1983, pp. 134–139.

Moyers, Bill. *Healing and the Mind.* New York, NY: Main Street Books, Doubleday, 1993.

"National Institute of Mental Health." *Medical World News.* January 1985, pp. 17, 20.

Pearson, Durk, and Sandy Shaw. *Life Extension.* New York: Warner Books, Inc., 1982.

Pelletier, Kenneth. Mind as Healer, Mind as Slayer. New York, NY: Dell Publishing Co., 1977.

Pert, Candace. *Molecules of Emotion.* New York: Scribner Publishing, 1997.

Pinchot, Roy B. (ed.) *The Brain—Mystery of Matter and Mind.* New York: Torstar Books, Inc., 1984.

Pines, Maya. "What You Eat Affects Your Brain." *Readers Digest.* September 1983, pp. 54–58.

Rapp, Doris. *Is This Your Child?* New York: Bantam Books, 1995.

Rately, John J. *A User's Guide to the Brain.* New York: Vintage Books, 2002.

Restak, Richard. *The Brain.* New York: Bantam Books, 1984.

Ricketts, Max, with Edwin Bien. *The Great Anxiety Escape.* La Mesa, CA: Matulungin Publishing, 1990.

Rogers, Sherry. *Pain Free in 6 Weeks.* Sarasota, FL: Sand Key Co, Inc., 2001.

Rogers, Sherry A., M.D. *Tired or Toxic?* Syracuse: Prestige Publishing, 1990.

Rogers, Sherry A., M.D. *Wellness Against All Odds.* Syracuse, NY: Prestige Publishing, 1994.

Roland, Per E. *Brain Activation.* New York, NY: Wiley-Liss, 1992.

Sahley, Billie J. *GABA, The Anxiety Amino Acid.* San Antonio: Pain & Stress Publications,[®] 2005.

Sahley, Billie J. and Katherine M. Birkner. *Heal with Amino Acids.* San Antonio: Pain & Stress Publications,[®] 2005.

Sahley, Billie J. *Post Trauma and Chronic Emotional Fatigue.* San Antonio, Texas: Pain & Stress Publications,[®] October 2002.

Sahley, Billie J. *Theanine, The Relaxation Amino Acid.* San Antonio, Texas: Pain & Stress Publications,[®] February 2004.

Sandler, M. et al. "Trace Amine Deficit In Depressive Illness: The Phenylalanine Connexion." *Acta Psychiatriaca Scandinavica Supplementation.* Vol. 280, 1980, pp. 29–39.

Shabert, Judy and Ehrlich, Nancy. *The Ultimate Nutrient Glutamine.* Garden City Park, NY: Avery Publishing Group, 1994.

Schatzberg, Alan F., and Charles B. Nemeroff. *Textbook of Psychopharmacology.* Washington, DC: American Psychiatric Press, Inc., 1995.

Schulick, Paul. *Ginger—Common Spice & Wonder Drug.* Brattleboro,VT: Herbal Free Press, Ltd., 1994.

Seyle, Hans. *Stress Without Distress.* New York: The New American Library, Inc., 1974, p. 36.

Slagle, Priscilla. *The Way Up From Down.* New York: St. Martin's Press, 1992.

Smith, Bernard H., and Antonio Rosich-Pla. "The Biochemistry of Mental Illness." *Psychosomatics.* April 1979, pp. 278–283.

Souba, Wiley. *Glutamine Physiology, Biochemistry and Nutrition in Critical Illness.* Austin, TX: R.G. Landes, 1993.

"Tracking the Chemistry of Stress." *Time.* June 6, 1983, p. 51.

Van Baak, Alice. "Tryptophan—Natural Alternative to Tranquilizers." *Bestways.* October 1981, pp. 63–64.

Vannice, Gretchen and Jill Kelly. "Mood Disorders and Omega-3 Fatty Acids." Nordic Naturals., 2004, pp. 1–5.

Whitaker, Julian. *Dr. Whitaker's Guide to Natural Healing.* Rocklin, CA: Prima Publishing, 1995.

Williams, Roger J. *Biochemical Individuality.* Austin, TX: University of Texas Press, 1979.

Williams, Roger J. and Kalita, Dwight K., eds. *A Physicians's Handbook on Orthomolecular Medicine.* New Canaan, CN: Keats Publishing, Inc., 1977.

Zucker, Martin. "Orthomolecular Psychiatry Update." *Let's Live Magazine.* November 1982, pp. 31–32.

Index

Addiction in America?
Prescription Medications

For every
prescription
drug, there
is a nutrient
that does the
same thing in
the brain!

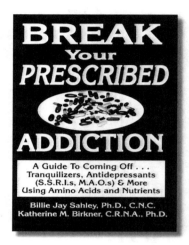

BREAK *Your* **PRESCRIBED ADDICTION**

A Guide To Coming Off . . .
Tranquilizers, Antidepressants
(S.S.R.I.s, M.A.O.s) & More
Using Amino Acids and Nutrients

Billie Jay Sahley, Ph.D., C.N.C.
Katherine M. Birkner, C.R.N.A., Ph.D.

- Finally, a step-by-step guide that outlines withdrawal and maintenance from prescription meds or addictive substances.

- Withdrawal schedules and amino acid and nutrient replacement programs included.

- Learn what amino acids and nutrients to use to withdraw safely.

- Answers for your questions regarding medications, natural replacements, and a proven natural approach to recovery.

- Learn why amino acids are so important to your health and by nourishing the brain and body you can successfully withdraw from drugs.

Break Your Prescribed Addiction $14.95

#1 Childhood and Adult Disorder is A.D.D.!

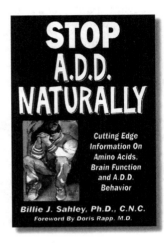

Learn to correct brain deficiencies and imbalances using the successful ortho-molecular program used at the Pain & Stress Center that has helped thousands of children and adults.

This approach is drug-free and puts back in brain what belongs there.

Follow the complete and easy-to-use guide that outlines the program including what to use, how much, and when.

Stop A.D.D. Naturally $9.95

Prescriptions for Ritalin have increased 2½ fold in the last 5 years.

If the trend continues, over 20 million children will be on Ritalin.

Ritalin is a stimulant and a Class II drug.

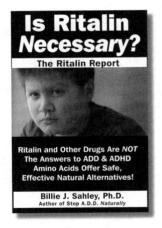

Learn about Ritalin and other drugs that are currently used to treat A.D.D.

This booklet is a must for parents, educators, and health care practitioners. It details information not only about Ritalin, but other addictive medications used for children.

Is Ritalin Necessary? The Ritalin Report $5

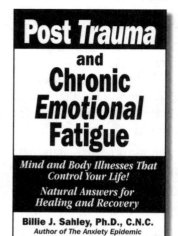
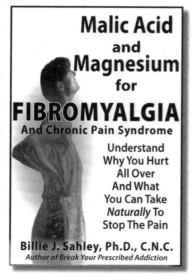

Reduce Your Stress and Protect Your Brain

Find out about Theanine, a new amino acid, that comes from green tea.

Lower stress and anxiety as theanine increases alpha waves in the brain without drowsiness.

This relaxes your muscles, reduces your tension, but does not cause drowsiness.

Learn how Theanine can change your mood.

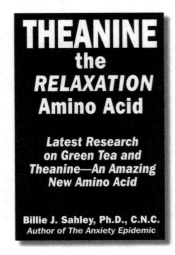

THEANINE
the
RELAXATION
Amino Acid

Latest Research on Green Tea and Theanine—An Amazing New Amino Acid

Billie J. Sahley, Ph.D., C.N.C.
Author of The Anxiety Epidemic

Theanine, The Relaxation Amino Acid $7.95

Fight Aging

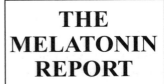

THE MELATONIN REPORT

How Melatonin Protects Your Brain
And Body Functions
Sleep-Wake Cycle
Seasonal Affective Disorder
and More

Billie J. Sahley, Ph.D.

Melatonin is a super antioxidant that decreases as we get older.

Melatonin influences hormones, neurotransmitters, and brain function.

Melatonin regulates our biological (circadian rhythm).

Learn why *Melatonin* is so important, who would benefit from it and who should not use *Melatonin*.

The Melatonin Report $3.95

Discover GABA

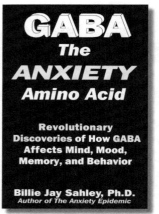

Now there is help for the millions addicted to prescription drugs for relief of anxiety. *Break* the grip of drugs, and *control* your anxiety *naturally!*

Find out why GABA . . .

- Controls the anxiety *stop switch.*
- Enables smooth functioning of both brains and enhanced brain functions.
- *Think* better and *feel* better *naturally.*

GABA, The Anxiety Amino Acid $8.95

Freedom from Alcohol Addiction

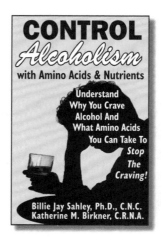

Alcoholism is a metabolic disorder that is treatable by balancing brain chemistry.

This book offers a safe, practical and effective nutrient program to help you overcome your craving.

Thousands have recovered using amino acids. This approach *puts back in your brain the nutrients that belong there!*

Control Alcoholism with Amino Acids and Nutrients $8.95

Protect Yourself Against Aging, Heart Disease, Cancer & More . . .

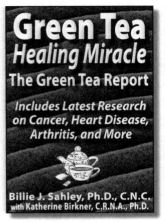

Green Tea
Healing Miracle
The Green Tea Report

Includes Latest Research on Cancer, Heart Disease, Arthritis, and More

Billie J. Sahley, Ph.D., C.N.C. with Katherine Birkner, C.R.N.A., Ph.D.

Finally, science is catching up with what Asians have known for years.

Numerous research studies document the amazing healing power of green tea.

Green tea possesses many properties to keep you healthy and fight aging.

Green tea helps prevent cancer and heart disease and protects against elevated cholesterol, brain aging, dental caries, weight gain, fights inflammation, and much more.

Green tea is a powerful antioxidant, antibacterial, and antivirus that supports your immune system effectively

The healing properties of Green Tea Extract offer a promise of healing that no other nutritional supplement can. The documented research behind this biochemical superstar has described Green Tea as possibly the most potent natural anti-cancer nutrient ever discovered.

- Stay young and healthy
- Fight disease and slow aging
- Enhance your immune system
- Prevent cancer and heart disease
- Reduce body weight
- Reduce your stress and promote sleep
- Protect yourself against bacteria and viruses

The long-term safety record of green tea is proven—and it is affordable for everyone!

Green Tea Healing Miracle $7.95

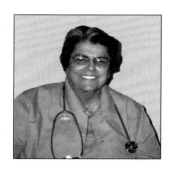

About the Author

Billie J. Sahley, Ph.D., is Executive Director of the Pain & Stress Center in San Antonio. She is a Board Certified Medical Psychotherapist & Psychodiagnostician, Board Certified Expert in Traumatic Stress Diplomate by American Academy of Experts in Traumatic Stress, Behavior Therapist, and an Orthomolecular Therapist. She is a Diplomate in the American Academy of Pain Management. Dr. Sahley is a graduate of the University of Texas, Clayton University School of Behavioral Medicine, and U.C.L.A. School of Integral Medicine. She is also a Certified Nutritional Consultant (C.N.C.). Additionally, she has studied advanced nutritional biochemistry through Jeffrey Bland, Ph.D. at Institute of Functional Medicine. She is a member of the Huxley Foundation/Academy of Orthomolecular Medicine, Academy of Psychosomatic Medicine, North American Nutrition and Preventive Medicine Association. In addition, she holds memberships in the Sports Medicine Foundation, American Association of Hypnotherapists, and American Mental Health Counselors Association. She also sits on the Scientific and Medical Advisory Board for Inter-Cal Corporation.

Dr. Sahley wrote: *Stop Hyperactivity/A.D.D. Naturally; GABA, the Anxiety Amino Acid; Malic Acid and Magnesium for Fibromyalgia and Chronic Pain Syndrome; Post Trauma and Chronic Emotional Fatigue; The Melatonin Report; Is Ritalin Necessary? The Ritalin Report; Theanine, the Relaxation Amino Acid;* and has recorded numerous audio cassette tapes and cds. She coauthored *Break Your Prescribed Addiction; Heal With Amino Acids, Control Alcoholism;* and *Green Tea Healing Miracle.*

In addition, Dr. Sahley holds three U.S. patents for: SAF, Calms Kids (SAF For Kids), and Anxiety Control 24. Dr. Sahley devotes the majority of her time to research, writing, and development of natural products to address brain deficiencies.